THE Mala Rubinstein Complete Beauty & Diet Book

THE Mala Rubinstein Complete Beauty & Diet Book

REVISED & UPDATED

Featuring The New Zig-Zag Diet

GROSSET & DUNLAP

PUBLISHERS   NEW YORK

Dedicated to women all over the world

Contents

My World in Beauty
and
How It Began

"Does it ever get to be routine—I mean, just like any other business?" a woman had asked me at a noisy cocktail party. It was the random fill-in that substitutes for conversation when the hubbub takes over. As it was asked, a waiter holding a tray of glasses above his head squeezed between us and at the same moment a man on my right, begging that I come and meet his wife, took my arm and steered me rather expertly to the other side of the room.

I never did find the first woman again to tell her "No—never, never!" Routine? Beauty? How could it ever be? Even apart from the beauty business, I find few "routine" things in life. Each grain in the sands of time differs from the other. Nothing is completely predictable. Our world is full of change, fraught with the unexpected. And of all its creatures, which is as varied, as unpredictable, as surprising as woman?

Capturing beauty for herself is every woman's goal. Sorting out the elements of beauty, shaping them and adapting them to the individual needs of millions of women has been my life-long vocation. It has been a constant challenge and a continuing education. Occasionally it has been frustrating, often it has been gratifying, but never, never has my work for beauty fallen into a dull pattern! A business that reflects a woman's demand for self-expression could never be static. The influences are as irresistible as the ocean's waves—fashion, moods of the times, local preferences, world events, even the seasons. And, of course, there is the "tidal wave" of scientific advance: A new ingredient, an improved method of formulation, an innovation in applicator or packaging can bring a radical change in presentation—and in results.

Beauty has existed as long as life. The business of beauty, however, is relatively new, and I feel I grew up with it. From my earliest childhood, I had a heroine who, in my eyes, outshone every fairy princess of fiction—my aunt, Helena Rubinstein. A pioneer of the cosmetic industry, she had started her own business in Australia, with more imagination than cash. After a stunning success, she arranged for one of her sisters in Poland to come to Melbourne to "mind the shop," while she moved on to new worlds and new markets. In dazzling succession she opened Salons in London and Paris, which drew the elegant and the famous. She crossed the Atlantic to start her American company. Her lines of endeavor seemed to reach everywhere.

Aunt Helena's letters and postcards reached us from every part of the globe. Her correspondence was newsy, frequent, and evinced an affectionate concern. She would ask about my school curriculum or if my tennis had improved—and I marveled that she found time to write so warmly when her own life was filled with consuming activity. Many of her beautiful photographs decorated the walls of our house, each whispering to me of the glamour of a world so different from the one I knew in Kraków, Poland. My life there revolved pleasantly around family gatherings, school, friends, Sunday picnics in the forest or a holiday excursion to the Salt Cave at Wieliczka. By the time I had reached my late teens, the future I envisioned for myself seesawed between two dreams: the practical one of being a housewife and the romantic one of being a poet. But, whether it was running a household or penning unforgettable prose, the *mise en scène* for my dream was always Kraków. The possibility of leaving that beautiful old city, with its medieval towers and buildings, and parting from my beloved family and friends, never occurred to me.

Then, toward the end of my last year at the academy, a letter arrived from Aunt Helena suggesting I come to visit her in Paris. Needless to say, the temptation was irresistible! An affirmative reply was sent and I immediately began planning my trip by taking what any young girl would consider the logical first step—I rushed to Florianska Street to buy a smart new outfit!

I will never forget the morning I left Kraków. In Poland at that time one didn't depart, even on a short holiday, without fanfare. My family and a multitude of friends were at the railroad station to see me off. There were flowers, jokes, advice, laughter, tears enough for a world voyage, much less a few weeks' vacation in Paris. Fortunately, the excitement and ceremony served to overshadow my nervousness. Before I knew it, I was waving good-by from the train and, even before Kraków disappeared from view, my terror at traveling alone for the first time, and to a country completely foreign to me, was almost forgotten as my thoughts leaped ahead to the adventure to come.

When I arrived in Paris, the city was drenched with brilliant sunshine. Riding from the station to my aunt's home on Faubourg Saint-Honoré, I was dazzled by the magnificent buildings, the wide boulevards, the elegance and grandeur, but I felt bewildered by the traffic, the number of people, the quicker pace. There was an urgency to which I had never been exposed. It was one to which I would soon become accustomed!

My aunt had planned a delightful holiday for me. There were excursions within Paris and outside the city.

Sometimes she would accompany me, but more often the demands on her time made this impossible. Occasionally, I was a silent, fascinated observer as I waited in her office, or followed her through the Salon or laboratory. Every day, Paris became more familiar. When I wasn't haunting the Louvre, I explored the many museums and galleries. Evenings I was introduced to a new, sophisticated world. Some nights I would absorb the stimulating conversation of the intellectuals, business associates, and many friends who seemed to converge on my aunt's apartment. Often we went to charming bistros. And, one unforgettable evening (this warranted a special bulletin home!) I made my first visit to the Folies-Bergère where the great Josephine Baker, then the toast of Paris, was performing.

My holiday rushed by as fast as the Parisians around me, but before I left my aunt hinted—so casually that I didn't take the thought seriously at the time—that someday I might be interested in working with her. After my return to Kraków, however, I was restless. The walls of my life there seemed to be closing in on me. In today's terms, I suppose I was striving for liberation. At the time, I felt only that I needed more scope, broader viewpoints, and the opportunity for constructive work. In an exchange of correspondence with my aunt, I offered myself as a novice willing to "try out" in the growing beauty business, and she accepted me "on trial."

When I moved to Paris, it was without any illusion of having a career offered to me on a silver platter. On the contrary, I knew that Helena Rubinstein, indefatigable herself, would expect from me more time, more toil, more dedication than she would ask of any nonrelated employee. Besides, I was determined to prove my own worth. During my "trial period" I knew my aunt was giving me the most rigorous test. The affectionate woman I knew as Aunt Helena in private life was Madame Rubinstein in business—and there was no overlap of roles. I survived the first few weeks and surmised that I had passed my test when plans were made for me to study with dermatologists in Vienna and later in Berlin. The studies were intensive but rewarding, and by the time I returned to France I had a sound foundation of basic knowledge that would be important to my work in the coming years.

Of course there was still much to learn. After my indoctrination, I started "from the bottom" in the Helena Rubinstein company, learning every facet of the business as I went along. I worked in the Salon, the office, the laboratory, the stores. Working ten and twelve hours a day, working through weekends, was to be expected. Many personal plans were sacrificed. Often I would be handed an assignment that others had refused; my aunt knew I wouldn't say no. The price of kinship was high—but the lessons I learned were invaluable.

If Madame Rubinstein was a demanding teacher, she was also a wise one. Observing her in business meetings, absorbing her love of challenge, following the clear-cut logic with which she solved what seemed to be insoluble, was a liberal education in itself. She loved to impart her business philosophy, and one of the first lessons she gave me was summed up in a single word: "listen." She was so right. I listened and then listened even more carefully to the message behind the words. The message behind the message sometimes! I listened and absorbed and learned. I'm still listening and still learning.

Traveling throughout Europe as a representative of the Helena Rubinstein firm was my next assignment. First I covered France—and learned that the Paris I had come to know quite well was quite different from the rest of the country. In the provinces, women prided themselves on their frugality. These were the days before broad advertising campaigns, big store promotions, publicity stunts. Many women outside of large cities were completely unfamiliar with commercial cosmetics—and they were skeptical. Some thought any makeup was frivolous. It was a challenge for me, after the fashionable Parisians who had a long tradition of beauty and not only desired but demanded the best in cosmetics. I learned that a more intimate, personal approach was necessary. By the time I moved on to other European countries I had learned to study the women of each locality first, to find what *their* own needs and demands were, to "listen" as Madame Rubinstein had so wisely counseled—and then to devise the best means of serving them.

Many thousands of miles and several years later, I was appointed manager of the Helena Rubinstein Salon in Paris. After my peripatetic life, I felt great luxury in being able to sink roots—to work and live in one city. The Salon was humming with activity and I hummed along with it. The world was in the swing of the '30s, and Paris was a magnet for writers, painters, sculptors, philosophers. I met the famous and famous-to-be. This was the time when my own interest in art was growing—an appreciation that would add a dimension of great pleasure to my life. Happily, I had met a charming man—Victor Silson—who shared this interest. Together we visited numerous galleries and enjoyed many of the fascinations of Paris. That beautiful city seemed to shine with new light!

One evening as I left the Salon after a busy day, any tiredness vanquished by anticipation of my date that evening, I thought—"How good my life is now. This is what I have waited and worked for." The next day my aunt called me into her office. "Mala, I would like you to go to America," she said. I am sure it seems strange to say I hesitated. A thousand people would have given anything to be in my shoes. But my shoes were so happily planted in Paris. I had my own home at last, my circle of friends, my colleagues at the Salon, clients whom I knew so well, the work I had built up, and the Salon of which I was so proud. Leave all this for another country where I knew absolutely no one? And a place so distant!

The Helena Rubinstein company in the United States had been established some years before. However, my aunt's attention was divided between many countries, and she wanted me to concentrate mine, at least for several years, on the United States. I hesitated, yes—but my sense of adventure finally prevailed. As I whispered, *"au revoir Paris,"* it was with every expectation of returning before long.

The crossing was rough. But every pitch and roll of the boat was well compensated for by the view as we sailed into New York Harbor. Today's jet travel is wonderfully convenient, but it does deprive the traveler of that magnificent first impression one gets from shipboard—the great size and welcoming attitude of the Statue of Liberty, the towering skyline of Manhattan, the bay that seems to wrap arriving vessels with a sheltering embrace. As I walked down the gangplank that snowy day in the winter of 1934, I indeed felt that I was entering a new world. At every turn there was something to marvel at in this compact wonderland. The snow-blanketed Central Park I viewed from my hotel window was as thrilling as the skyscrapers. I drank in New York as quickly as possible. After only two weeks there (and much of it inside the Helena Rubinstein offices) I left on a trip through the country that was to last two years. But what years they were to be!

First I discovered America—a land vaster, newer, completely different from any I had known. Here was a country with every kind of weather—torrid to frigid, desert arid to swampy damp; populated with people from every continent, of every ethnic origin. I felt like an explorer setting forth daily into the unknown! There was need for personal adjustment to the climate, language, food, customs. Even more important, I had to adapt my beauty knowledge for this new land. What had been so right for Europe didn't necessarily apply here.

I was introduced to the United States at an interesting time. The country was still working its way out of the Great

Depression. Money was scarce and spent judiciously. Travel was not as fast, simple, and available as it is today. Commercial air travel was in its inception and rarely used. Trains were the rule. However, for the average person, any and all pleasure trips were limited by the economic situation. Naturally, there was a great isolation of people in many areas. The restriction of thought to purely local interests was something unimaginable today, when even a recluse has the world brought into her living room through the magic of television.

Crisscrossing the country, I spoke with thousands of women to ensure my clear understanding of the American woman's needs, desires, and her own very special mystique. In some of the rural areas I visited, I felt like a rare bird watched through the binoculars of the most avid ornithologists! Women came to stores just to see what I looked like or to hear me speak. They were disarmingly direct in discussing their problems and frank in telling me they would buy what I recommended because I was obviously sincere and they respected the reputation of the company! In my contact with American women, I sensed immediately a mutual understanding and mutual appreciation.

I was concerned, however, with the amount of missionary work to be done. The American climate, on the whole, is much harsher on the complexion than the more temperate, damper clime of Europe. Yet American women, who apparently loved the great outdoors, gave their complexions neither the protection nor the restorative treatment that European women depended upon. I recognized the need for new products to serve the specific needs of the American woman—creams and lotions of lighter texture, quicker and easier to use, with greater moisturizing effect. Makeup, though more available and more widely used than skin-care products, was still rather limited. Generally, the range consisted of three shades: light, medium, and dark—despite the myriad color types among the many ethnic groups in the United States. Rouge was too dark, foundations and powder too heavy. There was an urgent need for education of the public in the use of cosmetics, the principles of beauty. As I realized the scope of the job to be done, I warmed to the challenge.

I began to feel very much at home in America. The joy I felt in my work, my surroundings, my new acquaintances, was enhanced, no doubt, by the fact that the good friend from whom I had been loath to part in Paris was now in the United States. Victor Silson's work had brought him to New York only a few months after my own arrival. How we managed to snatch time to meet each other here and there in these vast United States, despite our individual and quite different business schedules, can be considered one of love's triumphs over all! The difficulties of time and travel convinced us that the circumstances ruled out a protracted courtship and the obvious step was to marry as soon as possible. We set the date "between trips" and settled for a one-day honeymoon. As a follow-up, I became a citizen of the United States.

I continued my work as special emissary for Helena Rubinstein. Along with my travels and store promotions there were many projects—the development of new products and colors, the creation of special TV makeup when that medium was in its infancy, public relations plans. Cosmetics were becoming more sophisticated, more specialized; women were more knowledgeable in their use. The picture was constantly changing and my days were invariably exciting. In 1940 my aunt asked me to take the Helena Rubinstein Salons under my wing. There were several operating in large cities at that time.

Big, luxurious salons were then enjoying great popularity. I had always felt that they served a need—but a limited one. Artistically decorated, lavishly furnished, perfectly equipped, and staffed with specialists, they were indeed "beauty palaces" for women who had the time and the means to enjoy sybaritic pleasure and expert services. Many wealthy women came daily—for body massage, for facials, for private exercise sessions, to have their makeup applied, their nails manicured, their hair combed. But I thought about the millions of women who didn't have the time or the money for such pampering—and the women who did, but were so dependent on service from others that, left to their own devices, they couldn't cope with their own makeup, hair, or beauty. For a long time I had felt that teaching a woman to be her *own* beauty expert was more important than showering her with the most expert attention. Without diminishing the luxurious services of our Salons, I put increasing emphasis on lessons in skin care and makeup and developed "package plans" within reach of the average career girl.

My headquarters were in New York, and I was charged with creative development as well as Helena Rubinstein Salon operations when World War II started. I involved myself in War Bond drives. There was tremendous demand for grooming and beauty instruction from factories, offices, government agencies—all those institutions that had replaced manpower with womanpower. Many women had come out of retirement, or the kitchen, or other comfortable niches to handle vital work. Some found themselves competing, for the first time in years, for jobs, for status, for men! I gave lectures in airplane hangars, munitions plants, shipyards, and offices, and trained a staff to do similar work throughout the country.

To answer the need for beauty lessons, I organized classes at our Salons—head-to-toe instruction for women who had little time and not much money. Our five-day "Wonder School" was created. It was exciting to see the girls and women of every age, every métier, who filled the classes morning, afternoon, and evening. From lesson to lesson the improvement was apparent. Bodies straightened (good posture has been my first rule always!), complexions saw new daylight, makeup became more attractive. There was instruction in hair care, voice, diet, exercise, grooming, principles of fashion. The metamorphosis surprised many of the students, as they found themselves transformed into slimmer, prettier, more glamorous creatures. The effect on morale was tremendous. Many of the girls told me the classes had kept their spirits "flying" during the darkest hours.

Then I was requested to apply my knowledge to an urgent need. Many wounded servicemen who had been returned to hospitals in the United States would require plastic surgery, but the complete physical repair could not be accomplished at once. During the interim period and while the scars healed, there was need for expert camouflage makeup. This was deemed essential for the morale of the wounded man and for his family, too, to cushion the shock they might feel on seeing him again. I was asked to create the special makeup that was needed. I felt my heart twist and my throat constrict the first time I walked into a ward filled with badly disfigured young men. In each one I saw my younger brother who was then fighting in Europe. I knew I couldn't waver—that a display of emotion or sorrow was the last thing they needed. These were gallant men. As I worked with them, many joked about their "makeup," the new faces they would have one day. A sense of humor is often the banner flown by the stoutest heart.

The postwar years saw widening horizons in the cosmetic industry. The age of technology had dawned and, typically, life became more complicated. To me it seemed vitally important that neither our company thinking nor my own approach become too mechanical. Women were never meant to be fodder for computers! Despite the demands of business, I made time for direct contact with women. I talked with college groups, with teenagers, with women's service organizations. I have always felt that cosmetics have great therapeutic value. Psychologists and doctors know that interest in one's appearance often marks the turning point for a patient, whether her problem has been emotional or physical. I saw this demonstrated again and again as I developed grooming programs for the disturbed, the handicapped, the hospitalized.

Each year brought new fashions, new makeup "looks"—new products, and new shades to achieve them. Creativity and imagination became more essential than ever. I found, over and over again, that my interest in art, which had begun as pure pleasure during my youth in Paris, was an indispensable aid in my work. The excitement, color, spark, which I can experience from looking at a painting or sculpture is readily transferred to designing makeup. Subtle color gradation, line, form, are all there.

Along with the job of creating, there were many special projects. One I found of particular interest was organizing the Beauty Kiosk at the American National Exhibition at Sokolniki Park in Moscow in 1959. When Helena Rubinstein was first approached and the participation of her company requested, she had said, "I'll approve only if Mala takes charge of all our planning." So take charge I did. First I assembled a staff of beauty experts, all drawn from our Helena Rubinstein Salons. Each had to be a specialist in her area of beauty, fluent in Russian, unflappable under pressure, and politically acceptable to the Russian government. It was a tall order—but most adequately filled.

Russia had been firmly enclosed behind the Iron Curtain up to that time. We wondered what the reaction of the Russian people would be to the exhibition and to our part in it. As it turned out, our presentation was a "smash hit." The Beauty Kiosk was besieged by crowds of women, clamoring for the skin treatments and makeup services we were offering. The curiosity of the Russians was undisguised; their thirst for beauty boundless. Girls and women would arrive at the kiosk with gifts of flowers, cake, vodka. We couldn't cope with the number who begged for consultation or service. Some women received no more than a booklet (one had been especially prepared in the Russian language) or a tiny sample, yet even these were received with delight and many expressions of gratitude. The beauty demonstration that was given several times a day at our kiosk was shown throughout Sokolniki Park on closed circuit television. The monitors were as crowded and as closely watched as the live presentations. Madame Rubinstein came to Moscow for the opening of the exhibition. Her expression of great approval, after observing our Beauty Kiosk in operation, was a rare compliment.

Madame Helena Rubinstein continued to be active throughout her long, colorful life. She taught, inspired, and encouraged those of us who followed her. When she died in 1965, at the age of ninety-four, it was clear that the most fitting monument to her memory would be the continuation of her work for beauty. And it has gone on. My days are busier than ever, with more trips to every corner of the globe, more projects to be planned, more decisions to be made.

In the executive tower of the most thriving business, one can be enthroned in splendid isolation from the most important factor of all—the individual who is to be served. Towers and isolation I avoid like the plague. I try to meet and speak with women everywhere. How else can I be fully aware of their beauty interests, their beauty problems, and the best means of helping them? Each trip I make brings new interest, new zest, new inspiration. As I think of the count-less women I have met—in the Orient, in Europe, in Latin America, in the United States, in the Near East, the Middle East, every nook of our wide world—I am impressed anew with the unique individuality of human beings. How fasci-nating to find that each woman is distinctly *herself*—with her own dreams and aims, her own problems, and her own "private brand" of beauty!

Routine? The beauty business? Never—not in a thousand years! Exciting? Definitely—and it will be, until women are stamped out of the same mold and men stop looking. An impossible doomsday we'll never see!

For some time I have been urged by many people to assemble in one book all the basic beauty knowledge I have gathered over the years—in my studies, my work, my experience; knowledge I have imparted in personal meetings with women everywhere; knowledge that has formed the structure of courses for models, actresses, career girls, nurses, airline hostesses, and women in all walks of life; knowledge that, properly applied, can make the difference between ordinary and outstanding.

I have always said, "Someday—when I'm not so busy." I must concede, finally, that the not-so-busy "routine" day will never arrive. Why wait, then? There can be no better time than now to share with you my thoughts on beauty and my beauty ideas that will help *you* look your very best.

Approaching Beauty—
Good Isn't Good
Enough

When I was working at the Helena Rubinstein Salon in Paris, I lived in St. Cloud and spent my commuting hours doing a sort of beauty "homework." Each evening, from the time the train left Gare du Nord until it reached my station, I would analyze the appearance of the female passengers. The woman sitting across from me, I might decide, should lose twenty pounds. The one next to her has an interesting face but her hair style is too severe. The girl in the beret should do something about her oily skin. The blond would be stunning if only she would stand straight. What sallow skin on the woman in the purple coat! She needs to brighten her skintone and wear a pinker lipstick.

I had an abundant source of subjects. Mentally I would prescribe skin care and dream up a new makeup for each one. Still mentally, I would recommend steps for figure correction. And finally I would assemble for my subject a suitable wardrobe. If I found faults, it was only from an impersonal, professional standpoint. I was far happier, of course, when the subjects won top grades. There were many girls and women, hurrying home from a long day of work, sometimes in the simplest attire, who still displayed that incomparable French flair. Visually dissecting a truly attractive woman to define the elements most essential to her beauty was a rewarding exercise. The need for one's own style was obvious; a hairstyle, a hat, a lipstick shade that looked fantastically good on one woman might be all wrong on the woman standing next to her.

After considerable study (and many trips from Gare du Nord to St. Cloud!) I formed my beauty philosophy, which has changed little since then, and I would like to share it with you.

First, beauty is affirmative. It's what was *meant* to be, before the extra pounds, or the carelessness, or the wrong choice of fashion took over. With just a little effort most women can be far more beautiful than they are. Can *every* woman be beautiful? Yes, she can—in her own way. Every women cannot be Miss Universe or the most photographed model on two continents—but then every woman wouldn't want to. To be admired in one's own circle of friends, to be beautiful in the eyes of one's own children, or husband, or boyfriend or the man you'll meet tomorrow—is glory enough for most of us. And being satisfied with one's own reflection in the mirror gives self-confidence a hefty boost.

True beauty, beauty that lasts and looks good on grandmothers as well as teenagers, leans on the *basics*—clear skin, a well-toned figure, magnificent bearing, gleaming hair, an overall freshness. These are the timeless, built-in elements of beauty that once acquired can't merely be locked up for safekeeping. They must be worked for until achieved, then cultivated every day of one's life. The *fashion of beauty,* unlike the basics, is put on from day to day. It's ephemeral and lighthearted, yet no less important a part of attractiveness. Your own expression of contemporary awareness is reflected in your fashion of beauty—your hair style, your makeup, your clothes, and your attitude. Keep fashion in your beauty—or be labeled "last season's merchandise."

And then there is the *air of beauty.* It can't be measured and is difficult to define, but without it the basics and the fashion of beauty fall flat—if not dead. When I was attending the University of Kraków I had a schoolmate who was much admired. When Halka wore her hair in a plait, we all wanted to have plaits. When Halka pinned a rose on her dress, there was renewed interest in flowers. When Halka had her ears pierced, half the girls in the class followed suit. All of the female students didn't like Halka—far from it—but oh how they wished they could *be* like her!

By chance I met Halka in London many years later. A tall, handsome woman, groomed to perfection, moved gracefully across a theater lobby and took my hand in hers, "Mala, I'm Halka. Do you remember . . ." Of course, I could never forget Halka. Yet, as I looked at her with my now professionally analytical eye I was amazed to see that her features were not the divinely symmetrical ones I thought she had. Her eyes were set too close together, her nose was too long, her lips very thin. Yet none of this was conveyed in the overall impression.

We met the next day at Claridge's to reminisce over tea. After we had chatted for a time, Halka said, "Do you remember how gawky I was in school?" "Gawky? Why you were the prettiest girl in the class," I protested. Halka smilingly enumerated some of the physical imperfections I had noticed for the first time the night before. "And my height . . ." she added. "I towered over so many of the boys that I used to pray I would shrink a little!" She recalled that one evening, when she was shedding tears of nervousness before a holiday party and bemoaning her shortcomings her mother gave her firm advice: "Act as if you are beautiful, Halka, and everyone will think you are." Halka did act as if she was beautiful, and we thought she was beautiful—and she became beautiful. It was the air of beauty in action.

This same air has been put to work in many ways by many women. With some, it's a natural aura; others must nurture it a little. The air of beauty, to me, is an awareness of the heart and mind that complements one's physical aspect.

It starts within and works its way out, carrying along warmth and compassion and interest in others. It includes the inner whisper that reminds the body to stand tall, the mouth not to droop, the voice to be soft, the woman to be womanly.

In the train from Paris to St. Cloud I developed what I call my "look-twice look." I have used it ever since. When I look at a woman I see her two ways: first as she is in her visible physical state, and second (in my mind's eye) as she could be at her most affirmative, her very best. Sometimes the images are superimposed; the woman is making the most of her attributes; she has achieved her potential and elicits admiration. Often the images are far apart; in actual appearance the woman is a weed; she needs a lot of cultivation to bloom into the beauty she could be.

I advise every woman to develop a "look-twice look" herself. Practice by doing some people-watching. Oh yes, and please don't try it on your friends. You can't be as objective with them as you can with complete strangers. Besides, it is kinder to spare them your microscopic examination. Take a good look at women you see in the train, walking down the street, at any large gathering. Pick an individual at random and analyze her appearance for figure, carriage, hair, skin, fashion, overall impression. You can do it without obviously staring. As you "take apart" your subjects, notice what qualities make a woman instantly attractive; what spoils her appearance. Find, in those you analyze, examples to follow or avoid. After you have had a long, penetrating look at others, you'll be ready to see yourself with a "look-twice look"—the you of today, and the you you *can* be.

Surprisingly enough, few women have a clear picture of themselves as they really are. Over the years I have seen many woman earnestly groping for improvement but not quite grasping it because they were unaware of some obvious faults. One woman who always smiled at her reflection in the mirror didn't realize she wore a mournful expression in public. Another never smiled in the mirror; she didn't see the crooked teeth that spoiled her appearance for others. Some women carry a mental image of themselves as they appeared years before; some carry an image of how they would *like* to look and come to believe others see them that way; some prefer not to think about it at all. And very few women have that second picture of themselves—the mental image of what could be with a little more effort.

"Know thyself" applies to the appearance as well as the character. Unless you have complete, *correct* awareness of the present condition of your skin, hair, figure; unless you know the fashion effect created by your makeup, clothes, all your "put-ons"; unless you are sensitive to the impact you have on others—you have no starting point to work from. Only when you are searchingly honest in your self-analysis can you start moving in the right direction.

Once you really know yourself as you are, get your second self—the image of what you want to be—in focus. Be realistic about it. Your goal image must be suited to your age, your frame, and attributes. Try to visualize yourself at the ideal weight, with perfect posture, all basics in mint condition, every part of you polished and poised. Then decide how you are going to change the present you into the better you.

In any beauty course I organize, instructive charts and written records are part of the plan. I advise every woman to write out her *own* plan. You should start with a report on your vital statistics, head to toe, as they are today. Areas that need special attention should be noted. Your goal should be clearly defined. A progress chart, filled in periodically (monthly perhaps), serves to encourage your continued dedication as you record improvement in figure, skin, hair, every part of you that is on the way to being more attractive.

Plans are easier to follow when they're written down. Bridge builders, successful hostesses, businessmen, and great beauties can vouch for this. One of the world's most photographed models keeps what she refers to as her "Betterment Book." She clips from magazines exercises, diet tips, beauty ideas, and puts each in the correct section of her book. Sometimes she will add a photo of a hair style she may try when her hair grows longer, or fashion pictures that may influence her wardrobe planning for the coming season. She jots down a bit of philosophy occasionally, lists books she plans to read, even ideas for decorating and for entertaining. "I was a terribly disorganized person when I started modeling," she told me. "In this business, there's always someone younger—a new face—waiting to take your place. I knew I had to keep a step ahead to be better, so I started my Betterment Book."

Everyone mightn't have the time or inclination for such a detailed volume, but if you want to travel a fair distance along the way to beauty you will find even a brief record of great help. In the chapters to follow there will be information for you to fit into your own personal scheme. Jot down the points that relate specifically to your needs or, if you have one of those marvelous memories, keep them in your head. As you read along, keep in mind that your most effective tool is your own unswerving determination. Make up your mind, now and forever, that where your appearance is concerned, "good" is not good enough—"better" must be your aim, and don't be satisfied until you have reached the full potential of your radiant *best*.

1
Do You Know
Your Skin?

Many things go into the creation of a beautiful appearance, and one of the most important is a lovely complexion.

Ideals of beauty may vary from one generation to another. Fashions in "looks" change with the seasons. And then there is personal preference—"one man's meat" applies to more than the contents of his dinner plate! Women acclaimed as Great Beauties have been tall, short, fair, dark, blue- or brown-eyed. Beauty may come in every size, shape, color. But one unvarying prerequisite is a smooth, clear, fine-textured complexion. You can have the most perfect features in the world, but if your skin is bad, their appeal is diminished. On the other hand, I have known many women with asymmetrical features (and some with structural flaws!) whose petal-soft, radiant complexions have raised them far above the ordinary, won compliments, jobs, friends—yes, and the men they set their caps for!

I know from personal experience the great unhappiness a bad complexion can bring. When I was a teenager, attending school in Kraków, my skin suddenly "acted up." In my adolescence, antiblemish cosmetics were not readily available as they are today. Apart from inadequate remedies, the treatment was too often a "passing phase" shrug. Of course, we know now that *no* bad skin condition is a "passing phase." Actually it is a warning signal! Acne can leave pits and scars. An excessively oily skin invites enlarged pores. A dry skin is overly impressed by lines —and eventually furrows!

My own experience had a happy ending. My aunt, Helena Rubinstein, who pioneered the cosmetic industry, had been working with several European dermatologists and was already known for cosmetic products for blemished skin. Later these were to become the first treatments of their kind to be readily available at cosmetic counters. She visited Poland just when my "adolescent skin" was at its worst and—almost in the same breath as her greeting—prescribed specific care with some of her new products. They had to come from Paris and, while my first reaction was to shrug off my aunt's advice, by the time the package arrived I was impatient to try the contents. To my delight, I saw gradual but visible improvement in my skin condition.

Today a girl doesn't need an aunt in the cosmetics business. Whatever her skin condition or requirement, effective help is readily available. Whatever her age, she need not tolerate an imperfect complexion. Almost without exception, every woman can have a flawless complexion and retain it through the years. It can't be done by wishing, but it *can* be accomplished by following simple rules and devoting a few minutes every day to proper skin care. The time to start is *today*. It's never too soon. Early attention is not only corrective but preventive in its effect. And it's never too late. While neglect or abuse can leave a lasting imprint, I have personally seen remarkable improvement in the skins of women—young, not-so-young, and definitely mature—who conscientiously follow the skin-care regimes recommended for their specific needs.

WHAT IS THE SKIN?

The skin serves as a protective covering for the body. It breathes, it secretes vital fluids, it throws off waste. It contains blood vessels, lymphatics, nerves, nerve endings, hair follicles. There are actually seven layers that fall into one or another of the major categories: the epidermis, the dermis, and the subcutaneous tissue.

The epidermis is the outer surface—the part we see and touch. It is invisibly coated with a protective acid mantle and contains the pigmentation that determines the color of the complexion. However, the pores are its most important feature. Through these tiny openings the skin breathes, takes in nourishment and moisture, secretes necessary oils and expels harmful waste. One of the wonderful things about the skin is that it is constantly renewing itself. Invisibly but consistently the top layer is flaking. Dead cells form on it daily. They must be adequately cleansed away to avoid a flaky and lackluster look.

The dermis—middle area—contains the sebaceous glands which produce the vital skin oils and thus control the texture of the complexion. If they secrete too much oil, the pores enlarge and become susceptible to blemishes. If they secrete too little oil, the skin becomes dry, flaky, and is more vulnerable to external influences of climate and weather.

The subcutaneous tissue—deepest area—contains the sweat glands, the hair roots, the blood vessels, and nerves. It is from the subcutaneous tissue that the basic internal influences of the body are transmitted to the visible skin.

The skin is a complicated organism, intricate in its structure and function. Happily, it is responsive to good care—internal and external; it *is* self-renewing and remediable. And today every woman has within her reach the methods and means to make her complexion a beauty asset to be treasured lifelong.

WHAT'S GOOD FOR THE SKIN?

From time to time, women have begged me for a "magic formula"—some mysterious, secret ritual that would transform their skin overnight from not-so-good to radiant. There is no such thing! As we have seen, the skin is complex in its structure and many things contribute to its appearance. In listing some of the "good," however, I give first place to: *good health.* Care of the skin begins with care of oneself. Get sufficient sleep; most people function best on eight hours nightly. Exercise daily; it not only keeps the body toned and graceful, but encourages good blood circulation for a radiant complexion. Eat sensibly with accent on lean meats, fish, fresh fruits, raw and cooked vegetables, green salads. Drink plenty of water between meals. Be meticulous about *hygiene.* Fresh air is good for your complexion, but protect your skin against any harsh elements. *Emotional balance* is important for your skin. Happiness is best, if you can find it; otherwise, cultivate a philosophy that will bring peace of mind. *Love,* as well as making the world go 'round, puts a bloom on the complexion that no cosmetic can match! And, of great importance for the beauty of your skin—*regular care* with the cosmetic products recommended for your skin type.

WHAT'S BAD FOR THE SKIN?

The opposite of the "goods" are bad for your skin. *Poor health habits*—insufficient sleep, lack of exercise, improper eating habits. More fats and sugars than the body can burn up normally can lead to blackheads, whiteheads, pimples—especially in the very young. Too many stimulants, coffee, tea, or overspiced food are bad for many complexions, as are too many cigarettes. *Alcohol* taken in moderation won't harm, but don't overdo. That extra cocktail can leave puffiness, blotchiness. *The sun* can cause irreversible damage—premature aging; sagging, wrinkling, and discoloration of the skin, even skin cancer. Always apply an effective sunscreen before exposing your skin, and even then shade your face with a broad-brimmed hat. The fairer your skin, the more protection you need. *Too many pills,* unless on doctor's prescription, are bad. *Tension* is anathema, etching the wrong lines in the worst places! *Emotional upset* can leave its imprint in "breakouts" or dullness. *Negative attitudes* drag the whole face down and are so detrimental to the complexion that I urge you to stifle any such impulse before it takes shape. The worst enemy of all is *neglect*—neglect of one's health, neglect of one's philosophy, neglect of daily skin care. And neglect is inexcusable today. We know what makes the body tick—how to keep it ticking healthily. Wholesome foods are available to most people. Discipline can be cultivated. And as for daily skin care, modern cosmetics are more effective than ever, easier and simpler to use. A corrective, beauty-bringing skin-care routine can be as automatic as brushing the teeth—and take little more time. When good skin is yours for the having, why settle for less?

KNOW YOUR SKIN TYPE

Before you can plan your most effective skin regime, you must know your skin type. Do you know yours? Are you sure? Since the skin is under constant influence of diet, body chemistry, climate, the care you give it—and yes, even of time—its condition may have changed since you last "type cast" it. To determine your skin type *today,* cleanse your skin thoroughly. Place a magnifying mirror in a strong light and examine your skin texture closely. Check it against these skin-type descriptions:

NORMAL
This is the ideal—and rare! Fine-textured with no visible pores; smooth to the touch, without any look or feel of

oiliness. Most normal skin has a tendency to become more dry with time. The aim, in skin care, is to maintain its present balance and prevent the onset of flakiness or tiny lines.

DRY

There is a great prevalence of dry skin. It is generally fine-textured, but feels tightly drawn. It has a tendency to flake, chaps easily, and even at an early age may show tiny lines around the eyes and mouth. This type of skin is especially susceptible to dry indoor heat, air conditioning, wind, and sun. It should never be abused by too much soap and water. The lack of natural oils must be compensated by rich external lubrication.

SENSITIVE

Sensitive skin is dry skin "plus"! Fine-textured, often with a transparent look, the top layer is thinner, more sensitive. Tiny "spiderwebs" of broken capillaries sometimes appear on cheeks or nose. This skin reacts dramatically to both external and internal influences—sun, wind, emotions, certain foods. It cries for lubrication, protection, and "calming" skin care.

OILY

Overactive oil glands are the aggressors here, and the pores are fighting madly to throw off the excess. The result is a shiny surface, often a sallow look, and a tendency to enlarged pores. If the excess oil accumulates to clog the pores, blackheads and whiteheads become well-entrenched. The great need is to improve the skin's balance, to refine texture and prevent blemishes.

COMBINATION

Talk about inequity! In combination skin, nature delivers too much oil to the T zone (forehead, nose, inner cheeks, and chin)—but the rest of the face is shortchanged. Dryness is apparent around the eyes, the cheeks, the throat. Combination skin can be a minor or a major problem, depending on the degree of dryness and oiliness. The dry and oily conditions must be treated separately to keep the skin in perfect balance.

BLEMISHED SKIN

There's no difficulty in recognizing blemished skin! Unfortunately, it's all too obvious. Problems of acne and pimples are most apt to occur during adolescence, but are not necessarily confined to the young. Like mumps, acne sometimes strikes a telling blow at the more mature! Even an occasional pimple must be treated promptly to avoid infection—and to just get rid of the nasty thing. A more general blemished condition needs concentrated attention with medicated cosmetics that dry and heal.

OFF TO A GOOD START

Recognize your skin type? Now you are ready to plan the precise treatment it requires. First, just three rules that apply to *everyone.*

SELECT THE COSMETICS THAT ARE RIGHT FOR YOUR SKIN

Cosmetics today are especially designed for each specific complexion need. Yesterday's all-purpose cream, like yesteryear's patent medicine cure-all, has been replaced by scientific formulations containing new ingredients that have a singular target. Used for their express purpose, today's specialized cosmetics promise faster, more effective results. However, the finest cosmetic from the most advanced research laboratory cannot perform "miracles" if it is used on a skin type other than that for which it is created. Product A may work wonders for friend Marylou, but if your skin need is different, it may not be at all satisfactory for you. Be sure your time and money are invested in a cosmetic that is of a formulation geared to *your* complexion requirement.

PLAN YOUR OWN "SALON"

Decide on the one place where your beauty ritual will take place and equip it as efficiently and as prettily as a small "Salon." Whether it is your bathroom, dressing room, or bedroom, keep your beauty essentials in an easily accessible place. Line up jars and bottles in the order in which you use them. Keep all containers neat, smudge-free, and appealing! Have tissues and cotton close at hand. Include among the essentials a headband, to tie back and protect your hair whenever you are caring for your skin or applying makeup, and a plastic cape or makeup bib. When the atmosphere of your "beauty salon" is as pretty and feminine as you yourself, your daily program will be more enjoyable—and perhaps even more fruitful!

BE STEADFAST IN FOLLOWING YOUR DAILY SKIN CARE PROGRAM

The finest creams and lotions in the world—custom-planned for your skin—won't accomplish very much if you use them spasmodically. Important and lasting results come from consistent, day-in and day-out care. Set aside the time you need for beauty. It needn't be more than a few minutes morning and evening—but don't skip and don't stint. Your appearance is YOU to the world, and your appearance is *your* creation—the end product of the care you give yourself. As I said earlier, your complexion is one of the most important aspects of your physical beauty. Devoting even a short period of time *every day* to recommended skin care can put a most rewarding reflection in your mirror.

2

Custom Care for a Flawless Complexion

CUSTOM CARE FOR NORMAL SKIN

Normal skin has been referred to as a complexion condition "in transit"! It's almost too good to be true, especially today when so many disruptive influences tend to abrogate all normalcy—skinwise or otherwise!! Very often a normal skin is on its way to being dry—and less often it's heading for oiliness. If you are one of the fortunates whose skin is now in perfect balance, don't take it for granted. Obviously, it is easier to look after a healthy skin than to correct a problem, but don't be lulled into believing it will remain a thing of beauty forever without a little help from you. Every skin, like every plant in the garden, needs care. If it is not thoroughly and regularly cleansed, it will become coarsened. If it is not moisturized daily, there is a chance it will veer toward dryness. If you go on a fried-food binge, it might start oozing oil around the nose.

If your skin is normal (especially after twenty-five!) you must be doing something right—good genetic inheritance, sound health, proper diet, exercise, or whatever. Keep that up, and start your maintenance program of skin treatment right away. After all, your skin is precious—it deserves all the love you can lavish on it!

BASIC PROGRAM FOR NORMAL SKIN

IN THE MORNING

Cleanse with cream or lotion, applying with upward, outward motions. If you have a penchant for soap and water, this can be used instead. Be sure the soap is mild and the water tepid. Rinse several times to remove every last trace of soap.

Saturate a pad of cotton with mild skin freshener. Wipe it over the entire face and throat, using upward and outward strokes. Then pat the skin lightly for a feeling of refreshment.

Finish with moisturizing emulsion. It will protect under makeup and keep your skin dewy-soft and normal. Apply five dots—nose, chin, forehead, each cheek—and spread evenly over the entire face. Put a little on each of the index fingers and gently "fingerprint" around the eyes. Now take a little on the finger tips of both hands and with firm, long, sweeping strokes apply from collarbone to chin—left hand applying on right side of neck, right hand applying to left side of neck. Wait for the moisturizer to be completely absorbed before applying makeup.

MIDDAY

Cleanse, freshen, moisturize. If time does not permit complete cream cleansing, "quick-cleanse" with cotton pad saturated with skin freshener. Reapply moisturizing emulsion.

NIGHTTIME

Cleanse with cream or lotion. Tissue off. Repeat. (Soap and water does not dissolve and remove makeup as efficiently as a cleansing cream or cleansing lotion does. If you *must* use soap, remove makeup with cleansing cream *first*.)

Follow with skin freshener.

Apply moisturizing emulsion to maintain normal skin

balance. If the face has been exposed to wind, cold, or sun, use emollient night cream. Be sure to include the throat. After age twenty-five it may be advisable to use a night cream several times weekly.

"Fingerprint" eye cream in a circle around the eyes. This area shows first signs of dryness—here tiny laugh and squint lines are first imprinted. Early care provides the ounce of prevention that's well worth a few moments of time!

With good care and a good constitution your skin may retain its normal balance for life. As the trend in later years is toward dryness, however, do stay alert to signs and symptoms. Gradually adopt the dry-skin program, as the need arises, and keep your complexion lovely forever!

CUSTOM CARE FOR DRY SKIN

Generally fine-textured by nature, dry skin can be *very* pretty when it is treated intelligently. Obviously, it is hungry for moisture and lubrication, and what Nature doesn't provide abundantly enough from within, you can supplement with delightful, fast-absorbing creams and emulsions. Especially vulnerable in this skin type are the throat and the delicate tissue encircling the eyes. These are the areas where the least natural oil is secreted, and the first places to show signs of time, tension, neglect. Tiny lines become imprinted around the eyes; the throat takes on a crepey look. Prevention is the watchword, so the woman with dry skin is well-advised to start counteraction long before the first warning signal.

Be on guard against all deleterious influences. Sun can *really* be your undoing. Some of the most beautiful complexions I have seen belong to women who don't overexpose their faces to sun, wear broad-brimmed hats even on city streets, walk on the shady side, avoid the beach or tennis court during sunniest hours. You might find such discipline too restricting—or perhaps, as many do, you find the caress of the sun irresistible. If you can't resist, at least restrain. Limit your sunbathing; keep your body well-covered with sun lotion, your face slathered with protective sunscreen or sun-blocking agent. And *do* shade your face with a floppy hat or beach umbrella. You'll get enough color from reflected rays. Wind and cold are drying, too. Be sure your complexion is wearing its protective coat of moisturizer and oil-based foundation before you venture forth in winter. Artificial heat is another parching factor. If you spend many hours in an overheated room, a humidifier would be an excellent investment—for your beauty as well as your general well-being.

When I was new to the United States, on my first trip to the West, I saw many faces that were parched, lined, prematurely aged due to extreme dryness, while the rest of the anatomy was young and vital with health. What a vast difference I noticed on recent travels to the same "dry skin" states. Now the women of the West—who have always conveyed a very special image of beauty: confident, spirited, with a glow of outdoor living—have some of the smoothest, loveliest complexions in the world! In the intervening years, women there have met the demands of climate with concentrated treatment. Not everyone faces such challenging conditions, but how encouraging for every woman with dry skin that the right attention can bring such happy results.

BASIC PROGRAM FOR DRY SKIN
IN THE MORNING

Cleanse with cream or lotion formulated for dry skin. Apply with upward and outward strokes. Tissue off.

A splash of water is never enough in the morning. Haven't eight hours ticked by since your evening cleansing? During your sleep, the skin has been throwing off waste from inside the pores and catching microscopic air-borne dust, pollution, bacteria from outside. Morning cleansing whisks this away and gives the skin a clean, fresh start for the day.

After cleansing, saturate a pad of cotton with skin freshener for dry skin. Use same upward and outward strokes over entire throat and face, removing any last trace of cleanser. Now turn the cotton pad over and with the opposite side lightly pat the skin, moving upward and outward, for a feeling of tone and refreshment.

Finish with moisturizing emulsion. This will serve as a vital under-makeup protective and skin treatment. Apply five dots—nose, chin, forehead, each cheek—then spread it evenly over the entire face. Put a little on each of the index fingers and gently "fingerprint" around the eyes. Now take a little moisturizer on the fingertips of both hands and with long, sweeping strokes apply to the neck, from collarbone up to the chin. Wait for moisturizer to be thoroughly absorbed before applying makeup (you might clean your teeth in the meantime or complete some other small portion of your morning grooming).

MIDDAY

Cleanse, freshen, moisturize. If time does not permit complete cream cleansing, "quick-cleanse" with cotton pad saturated with skin freshener. Reapply moisturizing emulsion.

NIGHTTIME

Cleanse with cream or lotion formulated for dry skin. Tissue off. Reapply and tissue off. While today's cleansers are extremely efficient, this second application is important for completely removing every last trace of makeup and soil.

Follow with freshener, to leave the skin toned,

immaculate, and ready to gather the benefits of nighttime lubrication. Smooth on a rich emollient cream that will work deep to end skin dryness, applying all over the face with the exception of the eye area.

Pat eye cream around the eyes with gentle fingertip motions. Eye cream is rich in lubricants but extremely light in texture and designed especially for this delicate, dry-skin area. Only the smallest amount is needed and will be quickly absorbed. After ten minutes or so, blot up any surface residue with a tissue—again using a gentle patting motion—never pulling or stretching this delicate skin.

Always include your throat in your entire face treatment—cleansing, freshening, lubricating. Take some emollient night cream on the fingertips of both hands. Using the right hand, stroke firmly upward from collarbone to chin on the left side of the throat. Using the left hand, stroke firmly up the right side of the throat. Repeat these upward motions several times. Now, with the right hand held stiff, palm down, front side making contact, pat smartly under the chin, moving the hand back and forth from one end of the jawbone to the other as you make the brisk patting motions. When the throat calls for concentrated care, graduate from night cream to a specially formulated throat cream with firming plus lubricating action.

This is the basic program for dry-skin care, and I am sure your complexion will respond well to it. There are some "extras" which every skin requires from time to time—just as your body calls for an occasional tonic or vitamin to supplement your daily diet. Look for these under "Very Special Care for Very Special Beauty."

CUSTOM CARE FOR SENSITIVE SKIN

There is an enchantment in fragility—a tender flower, a butterfly's wing, a dew-dappled spider's web give inspiration to the poet. Sensitive skin has the same appealing delicacy, and—unfortunately—the same vulnerability. If your skin is sensitive, handle it as you would a priceless treasure—after all, that's what it is!

Since sensitive skin is extremely thin, it must be well-guarded against every harsh influence. Never expose it to direct rays of the sun; the immediate result can be drying, coarsening, and blotching. Long-range results can be disastrous—premature aging, wrinkling, uneven coloring, broken capillaries. Similar damage can result from severe cold or wind.

Sensitive skin needs *super* care and protection. In bitter cold or blustery weather, a second application of moisturizer (after the first has been thoroughly absorbed) is recommended as a protective shield under makeup. Sensitive skin often reacts unpleasantly to certain foods and fabrics. Try to determine the precursor of any little rash or irritation and avoid the culprit in the future.

Soap and water are *not* for the sensitive face. Light-textured face creams and soothing lotions are important—so is the technique of application. Take special care never to pull or stretch the skin. Since your body skin is delicate, too, use bath oil in the tub and after gently patting dry with a soft towel apply a body-smoothing lotion from toes to neck.

BASIC PROGRAM FOR SENSITIVE SKIN

IN THE MORNING

Cleanse—preferably with a gentle lotion cleanser or souffle-light cream—using careful upward and outward motions of fingertips. Don't pull or stretch the skin! Tissue off.

Saturate a pad of cotton with a gentle skin freshener. Choose one that contains no alcohol—perhaps one containing herbals or honey. Go over the entire face carefully, to remove any last trace of cleanser and to give a refreshed feeling. Smooth moisturizing emulsion over entire face and throat. It's important as an under-makeup treatment. Use gentle finger-patting motion around the eyes. Wait for the skin to "drink it in" (five minutes, while you complete the steps in your grooming)—then, if weather is harsh, reapply moisturizing emulsion to driest or most vulnerable facial areas.

MIDDAY

Repeat the morning routine if time allows. Otherwise, "quick-cleanse" with gentle skin freshener, smooth on moisturizing emulsion.

NIGHTTIME

Cleanse with gentle but deep-acting lotion or light-textured cream. Tissue off. Repeat. Be careful to avoid stretching the skin, especially around the eyes. Eye-makeup remover will whisk away all signs of liner, mascara, shadow, with minimum of pull or pressure.

Freshen with a gentle skin lotion.

Smooth on an emollient cream or beauty oil, upward and outward from chin across cheeks to temples, across the forehead.

"Fingerprint" eye cream gently around the eyes.

With both hands, stroke emollient cream or oil from collarbone to chin. Use light sweeping motions—upward only—with right hand applying cream to the left side of the throat; left hand applying to the right side. Pat under chin—from ear to ear—with back of the hand. Because of the great vulnerability of the sensitive skin, at an early age you will want to give it the extra pampering treatment of a throat cream with firming plus lubricating action.

One parting thought for the sensitive-skinned woman: Try to relax. This type of complexion reflects a sensitive nature. Your antenna is probably tuned in to the world's distress signals, and you can't answer *all* of them. Tension is quick to show on a sensitive skin—sometimes in blotches; sometimes in a drawn, aging look. You'll have to learn to break from its grip. Cultivate serenity. Lavish on your skin all the loving care it demands—and behold in your mirror a complexion of delicate beauty that will bring you compliments forever!

CUSTOM CARE FOR OILY SKIN

Looking on the bright side—oily skin is the least prone to show early signs of aging and is more resistant than dry skin to squint lines, crow's-feet, expression imprints. And that's the end of the bright side. On the shady side—along with a shiny nose—there is the threat of clogged pores, often leading to blackheads, whiteheads, and sometimes pimples.

A condition of extreme oiliness occurs most often in teens or early twenties—when the body chemistry is adjusting and the sebaceous glands are working overtime. However, some conditions will persist on into later years. At any age, skin that has been normal or even dry may become oily due to change in climate, or diet, or glandular action.

Whenever a girl comes to me with a problem of oiliness, I ask her to study her activities, her health, her emotions. Something is usually out of balance! If you want to clear up oiliness, start by being disciplined in your eating habits. Cut out fried foods, potato chips and other "nibbles," pastries, creamed dishes, rich sauces. Eat plenty of fresh fruits and vegetables, especially leafy greens. Salads are great if you can skip the dressing and substitute lemon juice. Limit the amount of butter or margarine you spread on your toast. Drink eight glasses of water daily between meals.

Watch your health generally. Get adequate sleep. Exercise (especially in the fresh air) induces good blood circulation, which helps the skin's balance. Hygiene is of great importance. Turbulence in one's emotional life can cause the skin's oil glands to act erratically. Although you can't program emotion out of your life, if you work on those influences that *can* be changed, you may find that problems of the spirit have dwindled along with worry about your complexion. Fortunately for every girl and woman, nearly all oily skin problems—major or minor—can be corrected and perfect skin balance restored through a program of specialized skin care.

BASIC PROGRAM FOR OILY SKIN
IN THE MORNING

Foam-wash with a deep-cleansing lotion. First wet your face with warm water, then take a small amount of the cleansing lotion between your two hands and massage it over your face with gentle circular motions. Give special attention to the corners of the nose, the inner cheeks, the chin, wherever the skin is oiliest. Rinse off thoroughly with warm water, finishing with tepid water. Pat dry with a spotlessly clean, soft towel.

Saturate a cotton pad with an astringent toning lotion. Choose one that will reduce oiliness while it helps tighten and refine the pores. Pat over the face, giving special attention to those areas where shine most often appears.

Next, smooth on, all over the face, one of the efficient new under-makeup treatments for oily skin. This will act as an invisible "face blotter" between your skin and your makeup, keeping oiliness in check for a long-lasting, no-shine look.

MIDDAY . . . A *must!!*

Repeat the complete morning treatment and reapply under-makeup treatment for oily skin.

NIGHTTIME

Foam-wash thoroughly to remove all makeup, soil, and excess oil from the pores.

Freshen with astringent lotion.

If the oily condition is extreme, smooth on a sparing amount of a special gel that helps blot up excess oils while you sleep.

Over twenty-five? . . . The throat and the area around the eyes may already show signs of dryness. These are vulnerable spots and preventive care is important. "Fingerprint" eye cream gently around the eyes. Use an emollient night cream or, better yet, throat cream from collarbone to chin. Apply with long, sweeping upward strokes, then pat firmly under the chin with back of the hand, moving from one end of the jawbone to the other with a smart patting motion.

TWICE WEEKLY

Treat your skin to a cleansing treatment "in depth" by using a friction-wash that cleans clogged pores with abrasive action. First moisten your face and hands with warm water. Then shake about a teaspoon of the cleansing granules into the palm of your hand. Work them up into a rich lather and apply to the face, massaging gently for just a few seconds. Concentrate on the clogged pores and blackheads. Rinse off thoroughly with warm, then tepid water.

Also twice weekly (but not on the same night you use friction-wash) . . . apply a facial mask that checks oiliness, tones the skin and gives a finer-textured look. Smooth it on over entire face, except for lips and area around eyes, leave it for ten minutes and then rinse off. Take a "quick mask" whenever you have a few minutes—applying it just to nose, cheeks, chin, or wherever oiliness is a problem.

Oily skin often means oily hair, since the scalp and skin interact. For the good of your complexion, as well as the appearance of your hair, use an efficient shampoo especially created to control this problem. Shampoo as often as needed—three times a week perhaps, reducing gradually as the condition is normalized.

Most oily skins will respond to the above program. Keep watching your mirror for beautiful developments! As the excessive oiliness is cleared up, phase out the oily-skin routine and phase in the normal-skin routine.

CUSTOM CARE FOR COMBINATION SKIN

If your skin is the combination type, it requires a little extra care, since you have two skin types on one face. What is good for one area is wrong for the other! Basically, you must use dry-skin treatment on the sides of the face, cheeks, eye area, throat—and the oily-skin treatment on the chin, nose, inner cheeks, center forehead.

BASIC PROGRAM FOR COMBINATION SKIN

IN THE MORNING

Cleanse thoroughly. If you're under twenty-five and dryness is not too acute, mild soap and water is permissible. Otherwise, use a cleansing cream and follow with skin freshener.

Saturate a cotton pad with an astringent pore lotion especially designed to correct oiliness and press this on the chin, nose, inner cheeks, center forehead—wherever the unwanted "greasy" look usually appears.

Smooth moisturizing emulsion over the dry areas of the face—cheeks, sides of face, eye area, throat.

If oiliness in the center panel of the face is excessive,

apply on this area under-makeup oily-skin treatment to act as a "face blotter" between your skin and your makeup, for a longer-lasting "no-shine" look. Always avoid using a lubricant on oily areas.

MIDDAY

Repeat the morning treatment. Or, if time does not allow, "quick-cleanse" with cotton pad saturated with skin freshener. Go over the oily areas with the astringent normalizing lotion. Reapply moisturizer on dry areas.

NIGHTTIME

Cleanse thoroughly with cleansing cream or lotion, to remove all makeup, soil, pollution, and excess oil. Repeat—or, if you are under twenty-five, follow with a mild soap-and-water wash.

Freshen and tone with skin freshener applied with cotton pad. Press astringent pore lotion on the oily areas.

Smooth emollient cream on the cheeks, upper lip, sides of face, throat. Apply eye cream around the eyes with gentle finger-patting motions. This is where you will first see signs of dryness, little crinkles that will change their name to wrinkles if you don't fend them off *early*. If you're very young, moisturizing emulsion may serve your dry-skin needs. Once you're beyond the debutante stage, however, give the dry areas the more intensive care of specialized products.

TWICE WEEKLY

After evening cleansing (and before freshening) wash away excess oiliness and help unclog pores with a friction-wash. First, moisten hands and face with warm water. Shake some of the cleansing granules into the palm of one hand. Work them up into a later and apply *to the oily area only,* massaging around the nose, inner cheeks, chin, center forehead for a minute or so. Rinse off thoroughly. Immediately apply emollient cream to dry areas.

Often, combination skin is a skin that is "going places" on the way to being more oily or more dry. With your consistent daily care, sound health habits, and meticulous hygiene it should arrive rather promptly at the right destination—Normal and Nice.

CUSTOM CARE FOR BLEMISHED SKIN

Problem Skin, Troubled Skin, Acne Skin, Teenage Skin—copywriters have devised a dozen names for it. Call it what you will, it's Heartbreak Skin to the one who has it. When does the villain of the piece strike? At almost any time of life. Most often the onset is during the teens when the body chemistry has to make terrific adjustment, and some skins don't clear the physiological hurdle too well. Sometimes emotional and physical factors combine to cause complexion flare-up. Sometimes the condition is fleeting; sometimes it is persistent. Whatever its status, when blemishes occur *act at once.* Blemishes shouldn't be tolerated for a moment. They can become infected. They can spread. They can lead to pitting and scarring that may permanently mar the complexion!

During my life in the beauty business, I have seen every degree of acne problem. I know from my own experience as well as from clinical observation of countless cases that there *can* be definite improvement, and there will be *if* the correct specialized skin treatment is combined with discipline in health and hygiene. Plan your campaign for clear skin and follow it religiously. Begin by tuning up your general health. Eight hours' sleep nightly, daily exercise, plenty of fresh air, are all "musts" for a good skin. Be a fanatic about cleanliness. Everything that touches your skin should be spotless—towels, pillowcases, finger-tips too! Shampoo your hair often enough to keep it free from excessive oiliness. A wholesome diet is extremely important. Here is my favorite food chart—for improved skin condition—and a wonderful feeling of well-being.

EAT YOUR WAY TO BEAUTY—AND A CLEAR COMPLEXION

Food not only fuels your body but also helps to form it! The right diet will put sparkle in your eyes, gleam in your hair, and beauty in your complexion.
Eat three meals daily at regular hours. Don't bolt your food; it's bad for your digestion and, eventually, your skin. A pleasant atmosphere and relaxed attitude are desirable!

EAT AND ENJOY Vegetables—raw or cooked
Lean meat (broiled, boiled, or roasted)
Fish (poached, broiled, or baked)
Leafy green salad (with lemon—no oil or vinegar)
Cottage cheese
Yogurt
Fresh fruit
Vegetable soup
Whole-grain cereal

EAT WITH MODERATION Bread (whole wheat, preferably)
Potatoes, rice, pasta, other starches
Cheese
Eggs (up to three a week—preferably poached)
Jello
Sherbet
Stewed fruit

DON'T EAT Fried food
Sausage and other spiced meats
Shellfish
Gravy
Cream sauce
Cake or pastry
Candy
Soft drinks
Alcoholic beverages

Go easy on coffee, tea, hot chocolate. Skim milk is a better choice! Don't nibble between meals—unless it's an apple, raw carrot, or celery stick.
Between meals drink at least eight glasses of water daily.

External treatment is of great importance. Medicated cosmetics will dry and heal eruptions, counteract oiliness to avoid further clogging of the pores, combat blackheads, and give a clearer, finer-textured look to the complexion. Be most conscientious in following your daily skin-care routine. There must be no skipping *ever* of any step until the blemished condition has been corrected.

BASIC PROGRAM FOR BLEMISHED SKIN

IN THE MORNING

Wash your hands thoroughly, moisten your face with warm running water, and wash with a medicated cleanser (don't use a washcloth—it can shelter the very bacteria that must be stamped out). Choose a liquid cleanser with ingredients that inhibit the growth of blemish-causing bacteria. Rinse thoroughly with clear running water. Pat dry with a clean soft towel.

Saturate a cotton pad with an astringent medicated lotion and gently press on over the entire face. This will freshen, reduce excess oiliness, and refine the texture of the skin.

Apply a medicated cream on all pimples. One that is greaseless and skin-tinted will not be obvious on the skin. This will work to dry and heal the pimples; also, by inhibiting the growth of bacteria, to prevent the spread of infection.

MIDDAY

Repeat the morning treatment if possible. Otherwise, "quick-cleanse" with the astringent medicated lotion and reapply the medicated cream on blemishes.

NIGHTTIME

Repeat the morning treatment. Sometimes there may be

some dry areas—throat, under eyes, sides of face—and appropriate moisturizing or lubricating preparation should be applied. Never apply an emollient cream to any blemished area!

TWICE WEEKLY

Deep-cleanse with a friction-wash to control blackheads and keep the pores free from clogging of excess oil. Wet the face with warm water. Pour about a teaspoonful of cleansing granules into the palm of one hand; add just enough water to work into a creamy foam. Apply to the face with fingertips, concentrating on blackheads and areas of excessive oiliness. Massage gently for a few seconds and rinse thoroughly.

Oiliness and blackheads can pose a problem on shoulders and back too. Use the cleansing granules to friction-wash this area when you are in the shower—and apply a healing medicated cream to any eruptions before dressing.

DID SOMEONE MENTION AGE?

We all have it—to greater or lesser degree. It isn't how much you have but what you do with it that counts.

Women who complain about their age are a terrible bore. Life offers many injustices, but you must admit it is very fair in dealing out ages. Everyone, but everyone, gets 365 days to a year. If you haven't used your years wisely or well, plan to do better for the future, and to be as attractive as you can today!

As for skin—I've seen some great-grandmothers with better complexions than many of their younger descendants—and I've seen the reverse too! The best insurance for a lovely skin in later years is correct, consistent care starting at an early age. But no skin is a lost cause. If you've been neglectful in the past, give extra attention starting right now. Follow instructions for your skin type—as shown on preceding pages. As time goes by, the glands send less oil and moisture to the surface and thus most skins become more dry. When Nature stints, give your skin the supplement of richer, more concentrated cosmetic emollients and moisturizers.

If you're over that certain age—or plan to be—turn to "A Question of Age," page 182, for some pertinent suggestions, which I hope you'll find helpful.

3

Very Special Care
for Very Special Beauty

That soupçon of extra effort makes all the difference between average and exciting—whether one is growing prize roses, designing hats, playing a concerto, or cooking a meal. Knowing where and how to add the extra-loving touch is the key to success in any métier. The same rule applies to creation of one's most attractive image. A little special care applied to your individual need can change your complexion from so-so to so-lovely! Let's consider a few of the truly desirable qualities of beauty that can be achieved through "bonus" attentions.

SUPERFINE-TEXTURED SKIN

Even the ancients recognized the value of facial "packs." Mud from the Nile Delta served many an Egyptian princess. Today, fortunately, there are sweeter, lovelier, and far more beneficial cosmetic masks! Their purpose is to firm and smooth the skin, refine the texture, and purge the pores. Along with all this, today's cosmetic masks give a stimulating "pick-up" to the skin while serving specialized needs.

DRY OR NORMAL SKIN?
Try a facial mask for smoothing, "brightening" effect.

DRY OR SENSITIVE SKIN?
Use a light-textured invisible mask that is gentle to the most delicate skin yet effectively smooths and firms.

OILY SKIN?
Use a normalizing mask to help correct oiliness and coarse pores while it smooths and gives a clearer look. This one can be used on the entire face or just on oily areas.

BLEMISHED SKIN?
A medicated mask will soothe and cool while counteracting excess oiliness and helping to heal eruptions.

At least once a week—before a special date or whenever your looks and spirits need a lift—use the mask treatment recommended for your skin type. First, tie your hair back and protect it with a headband or scarf. Be sure neck and shoulders are free and clear. Now smooth the mask on your face—upward and outward from chin to ears, from nose to temples, across forehead. Don't forget the space between upper lip and nose. The entire face should be covered except for lips and the area around the eyes. Keep mask at least one inch away from the eyes.

Take the phone off the hook, turn on some soft music, turn off all worries, and stretch out for ten or fifteen minutes. Try to keep a frownless, uplifted expression and dream blissful dreams as the facial mask is doing its beautiful work. Remove with a washcloth and tepid water. Then let your mirror and fingertips tell you how much this "extraloving touch" means to your complexion!

LIVELY-LOOKING RADIANCE
"My skin feels so lifeless," is a complaint I often hear. Dull, tired-looking skin, city-pallor skin, sallow skin need

help. Long ago, a famous dermatologist impressed upon me the relation of good blood circulation to healthy skin. It is blood that brings nourishment and life to the skin, that activates the complex working of the tissue. Good blood circulation clarifies and enlivens the skin, and is your complexion's very best friend!

If you play tennis, swim, jog, or get other active exercise daily, you probably have a natural radiance. However, some skins, despite all the physical activity that sends the blood cruising merrily, have a sallow look. Or there are days when everything goes wrong and you wind up feeling so thoroughly exhausted that even your face feels like it wants to sit down—and looks it, too! This is when outside help is in order, in the form of a cosmetic that lightly stimulates the surface of the skin for a lively look. A bracing lotion used in the morning, and any time after cleansing, gives a pleasant tingle. Saturate a cotton pad with it and pat over your throat and face (except the eye area) with a smart spanking motion. Also, a facial mask, especially the peel-off type, is definitely recommended as a "wake-up call" for tired-looking skin. As well as lightly stimulating, it helps slough off worn-out surface skin cells that can dull the skin. Use a mask at least once weekly, more often if you can, and always before an important evening. You'll relish the lively feeling as well as the radiant look it induces.

A YOUNG CONTOUR

How disconcerting for any woman, when her spirits are soaring, to find that her skin is starting to droop! Sag may be due to genetic factors, to drastic weight loss, to bad expression habits, or, alas, to time. If the condition is acute—if it is distressing or disadvantageous to one's career, love life, or ego—the logical solution is plastic surgery.

Fortunately, this isn't essential in most cases. Personally, I have always believed that the best way to fight time is by starting long before there is any sign of the enemy. Preventive care has won many victories and, at the very least, priceless delay. To preserve and attain firm facial contours, remember first your good-health rules and principles of basic skin care. Before the onset of sag, add to your beauty routine a firming and "lifting" treatment for the under-eye, laugh-line, jowl, and under-chin areas. A cosmetic "contour lift" is easy to use. Here's how it works.

AT NIGHT

After cleansing and freshening the skin, take a little of the contour product on fingertips. Using both hands, apply in firm upward strokes:

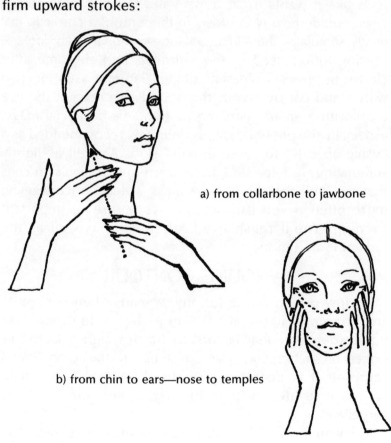

a) from collarbone to jawbone

b) from chin to ears—nose to temples

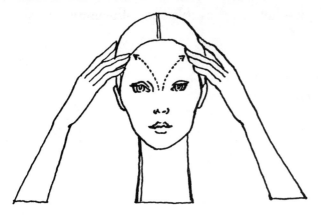

c) up between the eyes, over the forehead

d) *gently* under the eyes from outer corners to inner corners and out over the eyelids

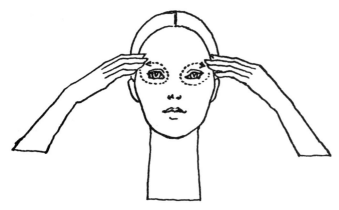

Now give flabby areas this special evening massage:

Chin

Use back of both hands and pat firmly under the chin, moving across from ear to ear with light slapping motion

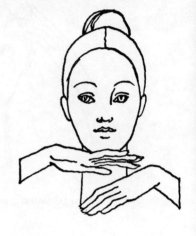

Jaw

Pat firmly, lifting upward in rhythmical 1-2-3 movement from jaw to temples

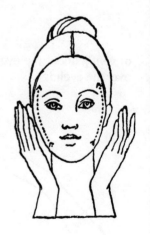

Inner Cheek

Puff out cheeks. Pat with finger tips along laugh lines, from corners of mouth up to nose

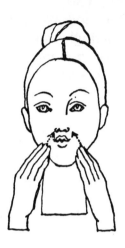

Under Eyes

"Play the piano," with quick little taps of your finger tips, moving from inner corners to outer corners, concentrating on little crows-feet at outside corners

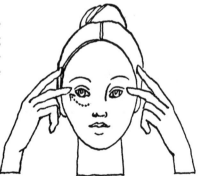

Be sure the contour treatment is thoroughly absorbed before applying night cream.

IN THE MORNING
Apply the contour treatment after cleansing and freshening, following instructions a, b, c, and d. Use it *very sparingly* and pat it in well. Wait until it is *thoroughly absorbed* and you feel its tightening action before applying moisturizer and makeup.

"FRENCH FACIAL GYMNASTICS"

"Facial Gymnastics" are fun to do and, if practiced daily, can help tone up the underlying muscle structure. You can do them whenever you have a few minutes (and privacy!) but for extra advantage exercise your face when it is thoroughly cleansed and wearing a rich emollient. Here are some of the "French Facial Gymnastics" which originated in our Paris Salon:

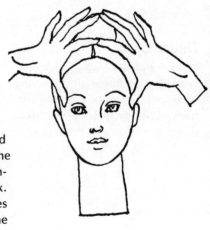

For Forehead
Make a half-circle of thumbs and forefingers on your head, above the hairline, with forefingers touching. Push back scalp and relax. Now try to make the scalp muscles contract up and back without the help of the fingers. Hold for count of six and relax. Repeat three to four times.

For Chin, Throat, and Jawline

With back straight, shoulders squared, drop the head back, letting the mouth fall open. With head back, *slowly* close the mouth, feeling the pull along your throat as you do. Purse lips in an exaggerated "kiss." Hold for count of three. Relax and bring head to normal position. Repeat several times.

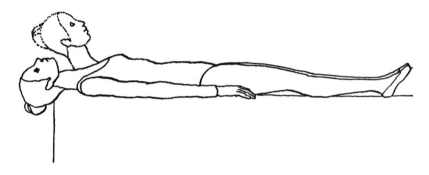

Lie across bed, head hanging over side. Lift head slowly, jaw thrust forward. Drop head back slowly. Repeat six to ten times.

For Cheek and Expression Lines

Press the three middle fingers of each hand underneath the cheekbones. Against the pressure of the fingers, smile in a forced manner. Hold for count of six and relax. Repeat two or three times.

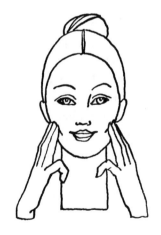

Purse the lips in tight kiss. Press closer and closer, making them as vertical in shape as possible. Now s-l-o-w-l-y unpurse and stretch the mouth widely open, as square as possible. (Say the word "W-O-W" slowly to yourself.) Come back, again very slowly, to pursed-lip position.

For Eye Area

Hold three fingers firmly at the outer corners of the eyes. Close eyes and blink hard, contracting the muscles around the eyes. Hold for count of six. Relax. Open eyes as wide as possible (without wrinkling forehead); hold for count of six and relax. Repeat two to three times.

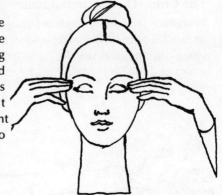

EYES IN THEIR BEST SETTING

Of course the eyes have it—and they tell it! They are the most *revealing* part of the anatomy. But is it always the *eyes* that speak—or the area around them? The delicate tissue surrounding the eyes is quick to show signs of strain, fatigue, neglect. This is the "setting" for your eyes and it must be treated with the greatest kindness. Since the way we use our eyes affects this fragile setting, an annual visit to the ophthalmologist is an important loving touch (and their due!). If glasses are prescribed, wear them! Frames can be chic fashion accessories. Today's contact lenses are easy to wear and more comfortable than ever. Even if you prefer framed glasses for general use, you might consider adding contacts to your eye wardrobe for occasions when you would rather show your eyes "unframed." Always use sun glasses in a strong glare. Choose them wisely; some prettily tinted lenses are not adequately protective. If your eyes have been strained by overlong reading or driving or wind or sun—give them this "refresher" break: shut the eyes and squeeze tight. Now relax all the muscles around the eyes, without opening them. Squeeze again. Relax. After repeating this several times, take two herbal eye pads, or saturate two pads of cotton with a mild skin freshener (preferably one which contains herbal ingredients). Stretch out (or lean back in a big chair) and place the pads over your eyes. Relax completely for ten to fifteen minutes. When time or place doesn't permit eye pads, try these "eye resters":

1. Gaze out of the window at the farthest point on the horizon. Focus on that distant spot for a minute or two. Now gradually draw in the focus—closer, slowly, closer.
2. Close your eyes. With elbows resting on a table or desk, gently "cup" the eyes with both palms curved over the lids. Don't press or squeeze; keep lids and eyes relaxed. Rest this way for two or three minutes.

Since the skin around the eyes is the most vulnerable of the entire body, in your skin care be careful never to stretch or pull it. Use a light-textured, emollient eye cream while you are young, before tiny lines become imprinted. The correct method for applying any eye cream or eye oil is with a light "fingerprinting." Tap it on all around the eye. Then "play the piano" with several fingers to "exercise" the area while the emollient is gently absorbed into the skin. Use it very sparingly; just a little goes a long, long way.

Puffiness under the eyes is generally due to an accumulation of body fluids caused by various physical factors. Eye strain could contribute—or insufficient sleep or too much sleep or sinus trouble or allergy. Puffy morning eyes are best alleviated by a cold compress (just wring a clean washcloth out of cold water and hold it firmly on the closed eyes for a few minutes). Follow with two minutes of the eye exercise shown on page 36. If the eye area is inclined to swell overnight, don't apply eye cream immediately before retiring. Instead, use it when you have an opportunity during the day—or at least one hour before bed, blotting off any surface residue before you turn in.

A "GRECIAN STATUE" THROAT

It has always amazed me that the throat—which should be as lovely as the sculptured marble of a Grecian statue—is sometimes the most neglected part of a woman's anatomy. One time when I was in Paris, a strikingly beautiful woman came to see me at our Salon there. She was swathed in furs practically to her ears and when she threw them off she instantly aged twenty years. A neglected throat marred her otherwise stunning appearance. It had brought her to seek professional advice (there was some whispering of a wandering husband), and in our conversation La Belle Dame repeated over and over that the lined, crepey condition had happened "overnight." Oddly enough, she really believed it! Of course, these things *don't* happen overnight. Too often a young woman takes her throat for granted, the not-so-young woman doesn't look at it closely enough—and the woman of a certain age hopes it is invisible! It's *not* and, like your eyes, your throat is a tattletale. If it tells the world you're older than you *are,* that's your fault.

Fortunately, I was able to help the Frenchwoman improve her throat (and, who knows?—maybe her love life!). The world's most beautiful throats—including some that have remained beautiful for decades—belong to women who have prized them and properly tended them every year along the way.

The first rule in my book for a good throat is good posture. Holding the neck straight, with the head high, will prevent many of the deep horizontal lines, the sag and droop, we see too frequently. When you are walking, don't thrust your head forward. Stretch your neck to the sky, and keep your chin parallel with the ground. At home, hold your book *up* when you are reading; don't press down on your chin to make it double! Check your sleeping habits. What about your sleeping posture? Sleeping without a pillow was grandmother's advice for a firm chin. If you can't manage that, at least use a *small* pillow. When you turn on your side is your head curled toward your chest? Straighten your neck; you'll sleep just as well!

Excess weight quickly finds its way to the neck, so watch those carbohydrates! Weight loss shows first in the same place! As with the body, the neck needs exercise to tone up the underlying muscles. Practice daily those shown on page 35 for "chin, throat, and jawline."

In maintaining your daily skin care, always include your throat. It's part of your complexion and part of the impression you convey to others.

The throat does not receive as much oil from the sebaceous glands as the face does. For this reason, it is finer-textured and less prone to blemishes—but far more vulnerable. Use cleansing cream and freshener on your throat just as you do on your face.

If the skin on the throat is normal, dry, or sensitive, use an emollient cream or oil nightly. Best of all is a throat treatment cream, formulated especially for this part of the anatomy, with firming, lubricating, and moisturizing ingredients. Use this same greaseless throat cream by day or, as an alternative, apply moisturizing emulsion.

Up is the direction of all applications on the throat. Hold the head high and starting from the collarbone, sweep upward on the left side of the throat with the right hand, the right side of the throat with the left hand. With the back of the right hand, pat firmly under the chin moving across from ear to ear.

If face treatment is for oily or blemished skin, carefully check your throat complexion. An oily throat is rare. Generally speaking, oily-skin treatment products—foam-wash, oil-arresting astringent, etc.—are best confined to the face, where the sebaceous glands are most active. Avoid using them on the throat. Usually mild soap and water (medicated soap if the skin is blemished) will suffice. Follow with a moisturizing emulsion—and if there are any pimples on the neck, touch them with a healing medicated cream. Even if the face is slightly oily, a light night cream or throat cream after evening cleansing is recommended.

A BANISHING OF SMALL FLAWS

Some "LITTLE THINGS" can loom large in the mirror and in one's worry center. They can often detract disproportionately from your attractiveness. In this chapter I will deal with those items related to the face that I am most frequently asked about.

MOLES

Most are harmless, but since they rarely contribute to one's attractiveness, why not ask your doctor about having them removed? He may do it himself or refer you to a dermatologist. It's simple and practically painless. The redness or small scab that follows removal generally will disappear in a week or so.

BROKEN CAPILLARIES

A dermatologist can drain the tiny veins with a special needle. But protect your skin to avoid recurrence!

UNWANTED HAIR

Off is the recommendation! But never, never use a razor on facial hair. A depilatory melts hair away below the surface so that growing-in time is longer and the regrowth finer. Choose one formulated especially for use on the face, and after hair removal apply a skin-smoothing cream. Electrolysis is the only permanent means of removing hair and is recommended for any coarse hairs on upper lip, chin, etc. Entrust electrolysis only to a qualified, specially trained technician! It is relatively expensive but a sound investment if facial hair is a problem. But *don't* extend it to your eyebrows! Fashions in brows change from time to time and you could wind up in permanent possession of an outdated expression. Depend on your tweezers for grooming and shaping brows except for hairs *between* the brows which may be permanently removed by electrolysis if you wish. Since light hair is less apparent than dark hair, bleaching is an alternative to removing facial hair. Use a bleach made especially for facial hair or have the job done at a reputable salon.

DISCOLORATIONS
Brown spots (so-called liver spots) are due to uneven distribution of pigment, an imbalance triggered by body chemistry. Sun encourages discoloration, so stay out of direct rays. Some spots can be removed by a planing process which should be done only by a most reliable dermatologist. You may find it adequate, however, to conceal discolorations with a skin-matching makeup created specifically for this purpose.

SKIN BLEACHING
Melanin, a factor within the skin tissue, determines its overall basic color, and there isn't much one can do to change it. Any bleach strong enough to drastically affect the skin color would be too harsh for comfort or safety. However, there are bleach and "lighten" creams available which help brighten darker complexions, fade freckles, or speed a departing suntan. Always patch-test a bleach product before using it on a large area and apply only on freshly cleansed skin. Don't expert miracles, but patient use may bring some visible lightening.

4

The Most Contemporary
Art—Makeup

The arts hold a fascination for all of us! What young
girl hasn't dreamed of dazzling success as a fashion
designer, best-selling novelist, prima ballerina, or movie
star? Unfortunately, the laurel leaf of fame is held out to a
rare few. But if the field for creative genius is limited, the
opportunity for creative expression is not. I am always
impressed by the women who channel their sense of
artistry significantly—not to reach the great anonymous
public, but to delight their own personal audiences. Decorating one's home invitingly, serving a gourmet meal,
planning a party or picnic with originality, composing a
verse for someone special, accomplishing any mundane
task with imagination—these are the creative arts for
today.

But the most practiced and perhaps most admired of
the contemporary arts is MAKEUP. I don't mean makeup
that one routinely "slips into" each morning, like lingerie—makeup that adds a little color, subtracts a little
shine, and does little else. I mean makeup that transforms
the appearance, defines the personality; that is, in short, an
artistic triumph for the wearer.

Just as there are various fashion styles, there are

many "looks" in makeup. Every women can develop skill in achieving the look that is most attractive for her. We hear a great deal about "The Natural Look." It's not to be confused with the unmade face. The Natural Look may require as many cosmetics, as much time, as much skill, as any other fashionable makeup. Its aim is to make the face appear as beautiful as one would *hope* to be "naturally," by simulating nature's own tones. Whether your beauty personality is best expressed by The Natural Look, or a more colorful fashion look, or one that leans toward charming feminine frivolity, today you can have at your fingertips everything you need to create your loveliest face.

If you appreciate fine art, you know how imaginatively the great masters have used light and shadow, tone on tone, color that leads the eye beyond reality to a more striking impression. The same principle of optical illusion is applied to contemporary makeup. It can be used not only to enhance and accent one's best features, but also to create distinct impressions. The observer's eye can be drawn to certain areas and away from others, without his even realizing it! Eyes can appear larger, or set further apart. The cheekbones and entire contour can be given a sculptured quality. The face that is too round or too long or too square can appear less so. With skillful makeup, every face—regardless of age or features—can appear more attractive, more interesting.

Women whose careers depend on their looks—models and actresses, for example—have learned how to use makeup to ultimate advantage. But *every* woman's face is her fortune, so to speak, and the one you display is *you* to the world. People can't turn you inside out to find if your heart is solid gold and your mind is pure poetry. "Face value" is often the basis for judgment—and if your face is its most attractive, fashionably dressed in up-to-the-minute makeup, your rating will be high. Every woman can be an expert with makeup—her *own* makeup artist—if she is interested enough to find the makeup shades that are most flattering and learn the method of application that best serves her individual needs. It takes just as long to apply a bad makeup as a good one, so why not master the technique of the creative makeup that turns ordinary into interesting, attractive into unforgettable?

BEFORE YOU START . . .

Decide what you wish to accomplish. Take a long, objective look at your face. Pretend your reflection in the mirror is a stranger, your mind the makeup artist. Scrutinize without mercy. Is the skintone good—does it need toning down or brightening? Are there shadows, discolorations, flaws to be concealed? Should the eyes be made to appear larger, or less prominent, more or less deep set? Do the brows frame most fittingly? Is the face shape too round, too long, too square, or just right? What is the best feature? What should be accented—and what minimized? What personality should be expressed—casual, romantic, dramatic, avant-garde? *You* are the artist about to create a special look for yourself, but you can't succeed unless you know what you must accomplish.

Create the right working atmosphere. We spoke earlier about the importance of creating one's own "salon" atmosphere for skin care. Now plan your makeup studio—perhaps in the very same spot. The first requirement, naturally, is a good mirror. If possible, it should be in direct daylight for applying day makeup. Otherwise, arrange for artificial lighting that closely simulates daylight and always check your finished makeup in a hand mirror *at the window* before you appear in public. The mirror should be well illuminated for applying evening makeup—we'll speak about night lights and their demands later on. Also, you'll need a magnifying mirror, especially for eye detail.

Headband to hold back your hair, plastic cape to protect clothing, cotton pads, and tissues should be at hand. No artist can produce a masterpiece without the right colors. Be sure your makeup palette has an adequate range of shades and materials.* Don't hold onto any unflattering shades because you want to "use them up." It's false economy. Today might be the most important day of your life—you can't afford to look less than your most attractive. Plan an orderly arrangement for your makeup items—an attractive box or tray. You should keep one complete set at your home "studio." A duplicate of any item needed for touch-up when you're away from home should be included in the cosmetic purse you carry in your handbag, in your desk at the office, or in your locker at the club.

Plan a practice session. Whatever the métier, before a great work is born considerable time goes into rehearsals, training, trial, and error. Set aside sufficient practice time for finding *your* perfect face. Try out various effects, different eye shapes, lip shapes, use of color. Be adventurous, but practice only in the privacy of your own "makeup studio" until you have mastered the technique and found the most attractive interpretation.

And always start with a clean complexion. That means cleansed and freshened immediately before applying makeup. From time to time, a woman will ask me, "Why should I cleanse my face in the morning?—I took off all my makeup just before bed." The answer, of course, is that while she slumbers her skin leads an active life. In the intervening hours, it picks up bacteria and invisible dust particles from the atmosphere and at the same time breathes out body waste (one of its functions), excess oil, perspiration. Whether it's morning, midday, evening, or

* There's a chart on page 47 showing basic requirements for day makeup, with additional cosmetics needed for correction and evening make-up.

bedtime, before applying makeup give your skin the thorough cleansing it needs. When you start with an immaculate surface your makeup will have a fresher, younger look—and your skin will stay healthier too.

BASIC STEPS FOR A BEAUTIFUL MAKEUP
I. UNDER-MAKEUP SKIN CARE

If your skin is normal or dry, apply a moisturizing emulsion to your freshly cleansed skin. It will serve as a beauty treatment *under* makeup, protecting against sun, wind, cold, keeping the skin dewy soft, and adding to the fresh appearance of the makeup to follow. First, apply to the throat, from collarbone to chin. Then dab five drops on the face—one on the nose, each cheek, chin, and forehead. Smooth upward and outward over the entire face, "fingerprinting" lightly around the eyes. Wait two to five minutes for the moisturizer to be completely absorbed before proceeding.

If your skin is oily, after cleansing and before makeup apply a normalizing product which forms an invisible "blotter" to prevent oil from seeping through and keeps makeup fresher looking for hours longer. This is smoothed over the entire face, if the oily condition is general, but not around the eyes or on the throat because these areas tend to be dry even when most of the face is not. If your skin is combination type, use the normalizing gel on oily areas only—nose, inner cheeks, chin, center of forehead—and apply moisturizing emulsion to the dry areas—sides of face, cheeks, eye area, throat.

2. MAKEUP BASE

This is the indispensable foundation for your makeup—for more reasons than one. It gives a smooth texture, evens out the skintone, often corrects or improves the

COSMETICS FOR BASIC MAKEUP

DAYTIME REQUIREMENTS	ADD FOR CORRECTION	ADD FOR EVENING
Undermakeup Moisturizing Emulsion (dry skin)		
or		
Premakeup Skin Normalizer (oily skin)		
Makeup Foundation—to match skintone	one lighter shade one darker shade shadow and flaw concealer	slightly warmer shade
Cheek Color		rosier tone or luminous glow-tone
Face Powder—to match skintone	translucent to blend over corrective foundation	slightly warmer shade
Eyebrow Makeup—pencil or blush-on		
Eye Shadow	2 or 3 shades neutrals for contouring white or highlight	brown or gray white or pale beige	frosted shades— one deeper tone
Eyeliner	basic shade	blue or green, if desired
Mascara	brown or black	blue or green, if desired
Lipstick	4 shades gloss stick	rosier shade and frosted brights

natural color, conceals small flaws, and helps the rest of your makeup to cling. And it also serves as a further protection against harsh elements of weather and pollution. Foundations come in many forms. For normal skin, young skin, travel convenience, there is makeup foundation in a stick. For dry skin, a liquid foundation with oil base. For sensitive skin, a souffle-textured cream foundation. For oily or blemished skin, a medicated foundation that helps dry up excess oiliness as it gives flattering coverage.

Choosing your foundation shade

Generally, the shade closest to your natural skintone is best. However, if your natural tone leaves something to be desired, a slight variance in foundation shade will help. When skin tends to be sallow, with a drab or lifeless look, a foundation with a touch of rosiness will give it a color pickup. The florid, flushed, or ruddy skin can be given a "cooled down" appearance with a soft beige tone. If the skin is overpale, especially if the hair is white or graying, the foundation should be just one shade deeper than skintone.

Applying foundation

If you are using cream or liquid, put a dot on the nose, each cheek, chin, forehead. If you are using a stick, put a small stroke in each of these places. Now blend the foundation over the entire face—upward and outward across the chin, over the cheeks, down the nose, under the nose tip, across the upper lip, across the forehead, *very* lightly around the eyes and over the lids. Be sure the entire face is covered evenly. Always use foundation sparingly. It's not meant to "mask" your face, but to enhance it.

3. SHADOW AND FLAW CONCEALER

Next step is to camouflage the "detractors"—those

shadows and flaws which may be relatively minor in themselves, but too often attract the observer's eye (when he should be noticing your *best* attributes). Detractors include dark shadows under the eyes or at the inner corners near the nose, "liver spots," coin-sized brown spots, birthmarks, dark moles, and other discolorations. If you have something to hide, you can do it with a concealing product—more opaque and with greater coverage than foundation. After applying foundation and before powdering, gently stroke the concealer on the area to be covered. Blend the edges carefully so that the camouflage is not apparent. If the flaw is small or not too intense in color (slight shadowing under the eyes or small scattering of broken capillaries, for example) choose a concealer that matches your natural skintone and your foundation. A flaw that is much lighter or much darker than your overall skin color will influence the shade of concealer used over it, and the shade must be adapted accordingly. To cover a reddish scar or birthmark intense in tone, use concealer one shade lighter than your natural skintone. To cover a lightened area, such as white scar or loss of pigment, use concealer one shade deeper than your natural skintone.

4. CHEEK COLOR

Light is the word. A sheer tint of color is all you need to brighten and define the cheek area. Just a little creates a wonderful impression of radiance and well-being, makes the eyes seem brighter and plays up their color, imparts a warmer look to the entire skintone. And just a little too much destroys the whole effect. So do use your cheek color with sparing artistry. Liquid, cream, or blusher stick are applied after foundation and before face powder. Cake blusher is applied after face powder. If skin is normal, dry, or combination, you can select any type cheek color you prefer. If skin is oily or blemished, cake blusher is preferable to other types.

Choosing your shade of cheek color

As a general rule, you might choose a cheek color of the same basic shade type as your foundation. If your skin is fair—a pink tone. Honey-warm skin, or the ruddy complexion—a peach tone. Medium-dark skin (or any complexion for a very natural look)—a tawny tone. Darker skin, to brighten sallow skin, and for use under night lights—rose tone.

Applying cheek color

Look in the mirror and visualize where your blush should be placed. To accent high cheekbones, and to create other special effects with cheek color, see "Reshaping" Your Face With Makeup.

- Start application on the cheekbone, at a point directly under the pupil of the eye (no closer than that to the nose) and sweep across the cheekbone, fading off at the sides of the face.
- Blush should extend no lower than the level of the nose (hold a pencil horizontally under your nose to check the area).
- Blush should extend no closer than one inch from the outer corner of the eye.
- Blend the edges carefully so that the eye can hardly tell where color starts or ends.

5. FACE POWDER

This important step "sets" your makeup and gives a finished, flawless look to the complexion. For the makeup that starts your day or your evening, I prefer loose powder. Compact powder is great for "touch-ups."

Choosing your face powder shade

Follow the same principle as with foundation—select the shade closest to your natural skintone. However, if your skin is sallow, choose face powder with an undertone of pink. If your skin is too ruddy, choose a more dun, beige shade. On oily skin, makeup takes on a darker sometimes "Orangey" look as the hours wear on and the excess oil seeps through; to avoid this, wear a shade slightly lighter than natural skintone—or translucent face powder, which gives a matte finish without adding color. Whatever the skin type, *translucent* is excellent for repowdering because it avoids the buildup of color.

Applying face powder

The puff you use is a matter of preference. It might be swansdown (my favorite), or velour, or a large piece of absorbent cotton. Just be sure it is always immaculate. If your skin is oily or blemished use absorbent cotton, replacing it frequently. Take a generous amount of face powder on your puff or cotton pad. Starting at the chin, apply upward with gentle pressing motions, covering the entire face—chin, cheeks, nose, eyes, forehead. Now—with the reverse side of your puff or another piece of cotton —gently dust across forehead and *down* cheeks, nose, chin, to flatten the very light, all-but-invisible downy hair on the surface. As a final touch, a soft complexion brush will whisk away any excess from around the eyes, at the corners of the nose, in laugh lines.

6. EYEBROWS

If the eyes have a language all their own, thank the brows for some of their most charming conversation. Eyebrows give expression and character to the face. Most brows come well shaped to frame the eyes below them, and while they may need grooming and definition think twice before you attempt to alter the basic form. Eyebrows can be rather temperamental—once banished they may never come back. I remember the craze for hairline-thin brows during the '30s and the bitter tears of some women who shaved or plucked in haste and were left with permanently outdated expressions.

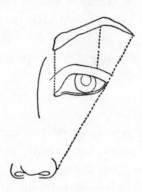

Ideally, the brow should start at a point over the inner corner of the eye, with the highest arch above the outer part of the iris. Hold a pencil in a slanting line from outer nostril, crossing the outer corner of the eye, to the brow. This will give you the right terminal point. Now hold the pencil horizontally under the brow. The end of the brow should never be lower than the beginning. Hairs between the brows should be plucked out, as well as any stragglers beneath the natural brow line. Before tweezing, cleanse the eyebrow area and apply a little lubricating cream to soften the skin. Be sure your tweezers are absolutely clean; dip them in alcohol before using. Tweeze with a quick, firm pull in the same direction as hair growth. After tweezing, wipe the area with a cotton pad saturated with astringent.

To define your brows you can use pencil or brush-on powder. Pencil gives a more definite effect and is preferable for shaping and filling in the brows. Brush-on eyebrow makeup gives a young look and is good for subtly coloring the brow without adding width or length.

Choosing your eyebrow makeup shade
Eyebrow makeup generally looks darker on the brow.

Unless your brows are very pale, choose a tone slightly lighter than your natural eyebrow color but one that will blend in attractively. Dark brown is preferable to black on all but the most dramatic brunettes. Light brown is good for brownettes, dark blonds, some redheads. Charcoal for the gray-haired and silvery blonds; ash blond for light blonds and pale redheads; and auburn or brown for dark redheads.

Applying eyebrow makeup

Brush the brows to remove any trace of powder. Now brush straight up, then across, to smooth the hairs in place. Apply eyebrow pencil in light, tiny lines, each one simulating a hair. (Be sure the pencil has a sharp point. A heavy line is never attractive.) Most brows need to be extended slightly at the end; be sure this line doesn't curve downward. The slightest lift at the outer end can give an uplifted expression. If you wish, brush again *very lightly* to blend the color evenly.

Brush-on eyebrow makeup is applied with the tip of the brush, making short, feathery strokes to add color where needed.

NOTE: If you have lightened your hair, perhaps your brows should be bleached. Or if your brows are pale to the point of oblivion, you may want to have them dyed. Neither one is a do-it-yourself job! Bleaches and dyes are potentially dangerous when used so close to the eyes. Leave them in the hands of a professional at a reputable beauty salon.

7. EYE SHADOW

Is there an artist in you, struggling to express herself? Now is your chance! Ask any model or actress. If she had to single out one makeup step that gives life to her looks, it would be her eye shadow. The miracles it performs are often unsung; cleverly applied it gives all credit to the eyes themselves—accenting their color and brilliance, contouring the bone area, creating fascinating optical illusions, giving new expression and appeal. By day, eye shadow should suit your face and the occasion. For a conservative look, you might choose neutral tones or subtle pastels. Whatever your daytime interpretation—understated, fashion accent, or "natural" look—shadow takes away that washed-out appearance of undressed lids, wakes up your eyes, makes your entire face seem more vibrant. For evening, your eye shadow should be more definitive. Choose stronger colors or luminous shades, which—subtly reflecting night lights—add glamour and sparkle. Using eye shadow effectively is often the difference between success and failure in achieving one's most attractive look. Never underestimate its importance to *your* beauty.

Eye shadow comes in several forms. Matte or powder shadow gives a soft, subtle look and is long-wearing on the lid. Cream shadow gives more highlight and gleam. There are forms in between—powdery creams and creamy powders. Choose the type you find most satisfactory for the specific "look" you want to achieve. You may like the effect of two textures: a matte shadow on the lid itself, a creamy one on the bone area. There are many possibilities for you to explore and enjoy.

Choosing your eye shadows
The well-dressed eye has a wardrobe of eye shadows. You will want one to match the color of your eyes: blue or soft green or copper—another to accent them by contrast: turquoise or violet or silvery gray. You should have fashionable tones to complement your favorite costume colors: lime or lilac or even pink. For contouring the eye area and creating exciting impressions you will need dark and light neutrals: taupe or brown to give a feeling of depth, pale beige or pearly white to highlight.

Applying your eye shadow
Matte eye shadow is stroked on with sponge-tip applicator. Cream eye shadow is smoothed on with the fingertip.

Shadow in stick form may be stroked on directly and the color then blended with the finger tip.

Always remember—light color makes an area appear more prominent; it seems to "come forward." Dark color makes an area seem less prominent; to "recede." If no corrective contouring is needed, choose a flattering shade and apply it on the eyelid, sweeping up and outward, lifting it at the end of the lid so that it fades off in the direction of the eyebrow's end. Use a neutral tone—darker than natural skintone (brown, taupe, or gray for example) on any area you want to "recede" such as heavy or puffy lid, or too prominent bone between the lid and the brow. Use a light tone—paler than skin color, on any area you want to bring forward; the eyelid itself if eyes are small or deep set or the brow bone if eyes are too prominent. A thin line of highlight just under the eyebrow, blended in gently with the fingertip, "opens up" and enhancces most eyes. On pages 66–67 you'll find complete instructions for optical illusions that "reshape" the eyes to new loveliness! Follow the directions that apply to *your* eyes. And on page 70 there are suggestions for the glamorous evening eye.

8. EYELINER

An important accent for the eye, liner helps define their shape, adds sparkle, and is a real "eye opener." Eyeliner comes in cake, liquid, and pencil form.

Choosing your eyeliner shade

Too dark a line will give a harsh look and draw attention away from the eye itself—which, after all, is the feature to spotlight. Use black eyeliner only if you have jet hair and dark skin. Dark brown is deep enough for most brunettes. Brownettes, blondes, redheads get flattering effects with taupe or soft brown tones. Charcoal gray looks good on many women, not only the gray-haired or silver blondes. Blue and green are good fashion accents; lovely for evening and for special daytime effect.

Applying eyeliner

Cake or liquid liner is applied with a fine-tipped brush. To draw a clean line more easily, look *down* into a magnifying mirror. With one finger at the outer corner of the eye, holding the lid taut, start at the inner corner and draw a thin line along the lid, as close to the lashes as possible, ending at the outer corner. If the eyes are too close together, start the liner about a quarter of an inch in from inner corner or at a point just above the inner iris and extend it a little beyond the outer end of the lid. Most women should use liner on the upper lid *only.* A line around the bottom of the eye closes it in; makes small and deep-set eyes seem more so, emphasizes any lines, shadows, or puffiness under the eye. If you are one of the few who *can* use liner under the eye, keep the line thin and just *under* the lashes (not over them).

Eyelining pencil is applied in basically the same manner. It doesn't give as sharp or lasting a line as cake or liquid; however, it is excellent for subtle effect. Also, if a softened "smudged" look is your fashion, you can accomplish this more easily with pencil. Just pat the line with your fingertip after applying.

9. MASCARA

Years ago, as I left a London cinema (yes, it was a *very* sad film) I was struck by the number of women who had little black smudges, and sometimes rivulets, wandering down their cheeks. I wondered if I was similarly marked and felt grateful, for once, for the dense London fog! Today, after the weepiest session, the longest walk in the rain, or even a swim, we can be grateful for mascara that stays in place, doesn't rub off or run off—and does such beguiling things for the eyes!

Beautiful lashes *do* frame the eyes in beauty, as they give a completely feminine and delightful look. And as lashes are rarely long enough or dark enough to win

compliments on their own, mascara is an everyday necessity for most women.

Mascara comes in several forms: cake, for most subtle
accent, liquid for more definition, waterproof cream mascara in tube for great convenience. My favorite is the
lash-building mascara that comes in a slim tube with its
own wand applicator. It has tiny filaments that cling to
your own lashes to actually make them thicker, lusher,
longer, as it adds color.

Choosing your mascara shade

Black for the raven-haired; dark brown for the brunette;
brown for brownettes, dark blondes, dark redheads; light
brown for blondes, fair redheads, graying hair; blue and
green can be dramatic on the right eyes but look best under
artificial light—save these colors for evening or apply them
to the tips *only* after using a conventional shade on the
entire lash.

Applying mascara

An automatic applicator is easiest to use. Each time you
draw the wand from the case it will hold the correct amount
of mascara for one eye. Hold the wand horizontal to the eye
(never turn the point toward the eye) and with a light,
lifting motion stroke upward from the roots of the lashes to
the tips. Wait a few seconds for the first application to dry,
then repeat.

If you use a brush for application, be careful not to
take too much mascara on it at one time. Two or even three
light applications are better than one heavy, lumpy one.
Take the mascara on the *side* of the brush; hold the brush
with the *sides* of the bristles facing your eye and brush
lightly upward, giving the brush a little twist so that as you
finish coloring the lash tips the bristles of the brush are
facing upward. Wait for the mascara to dry, then repeat the
application.

10. ARTIFICIAL LASHES

If your own lashes are sparse, or if you just want quickly to add a lush fringe, get yourself a pair of artificial lashes. From the variety of styles available, choose the one that suits your face and your lifestyle. Use the same rule for shade as you do for selecting mascara: Black for the darkest brunette only; brown for most brunettes, dark blondes and red-heads; ash for the very fair or silver-haired.

11. LIPSTICK

If lipsticks were as rare and costly as diamonds, which would rate as a girl's best friend? A hypothetical question—fortunately—doesn't need an answer, but actually I think it's nice to have both! Diamonds are beautiful to look at (yes—they have value too!); lipstick makes *you* beautiful to behold (and you're priceless, aren't you?). Lipstick is truly the indispensable makeup item. Just consider all it does for you. It colors your lips, makes your face come alive, accents your personal coloring, gives harmony to your fashion. It's a beauty treatment for your lips, protecting this delicate tissue from the parching effect of sun, wind and cold. And beyond that—it's part of the feminine mystique! Lipstick is a woman's ever-present talisman. In life's darkest moments, out comes the case and on goes the color—in a symbolic act of faith or hope or morale-building. In wartime, I've seen lipstick worn as a red badge of courage. In hospitals, I've witnessed the "turn for the better" when the patient suddenly demanded her lipstick. I've watched friends, crushed by emotional blows, finally dry their tears, square their shoulders—and reach for their lip color. But, most of all, I've seen it add brightness and glamour to all the waking hours of every day.

Only a woman knows (it surpasses male understanding!) the vital role lipstick plays in her life. She selects her lipsticks with care, considering both shade and texture. Too dry a texture will cause lips to flake, color to "roll." Too creamy a texture disappears too quickly and leaves its telltale imprints along the way. The perfect lipstick contains enough emollient to keep lips smooth and inviting—yet stays color-true until it is removed.

Selecting your lipstick colors

Everyone needs a wardrobe of lipstick shades—colors to complement skintone, hair, eyes; to harmonize with favorite fashion colors; to add an attractive accent in sunlight, candlelight, and all the lights in between! The depth of tone you select will depend on your personal coloring and on the current fashion (and the pendulum swings back and forth with great regularity!). Every woman should have a minimum of four shades in her lipstick wardrobe:

>a red tone
>a coral or peach
>a pink or rose
>a tawny beige or brown

Each can be worn alone—or one may be worn over another for a variety of tones and effects. Pink over peach, for example, with pastels—the tawny lipstick over red with beige or tan tweeds—rose over coral with a blue chiffon evening dress. Or outline in one shade and fill in with another. The possibilities and scope for your inventiveness are endless. Lip gloss gives high shine and light transparent color. It's often a teenager's first makeup but belongs in every woman's beauty wardrobe. Wear it alone for a young and natural look, for protecting and moisturizing, or for pretty bedtime lips. Wear it *under* conventional lipstick for extra lubrication when lips feel extremely dry. Wear it *over* lipstick for wet-looking shine.

Applying your lipstick

It isn't always practical when you're retouching during the day, but whenever possible (certainly whenever you do a complete makeup job) apply lipstick to clean lips. Use cream cleanser and tissue, being careful to remove *all* the cream. If you leave a residue of cream, your lipstick won't wear well.

With elbow resting on table for greater control, outline the bottom lip—from center to right corner, from center to left corner. Outline the upper lip from center to right corner, from center to left corner. Now fill in with color. Open the mouth to fill in lightly at the ends, being careful not to run over the lip line.

If natural lip shape is to be outlined, a base of foundation and powder is not needed. If the lip shape needs correction, include the lips when you apply makeup foundation and face powder. If the mouth is too large, outline just *inside* the natural line, using a light shade. Fill in with a slightly deeper but still relatively light shade. If the lips are too thin, outline in a light shade just *outside* the natural lip line and fill in with a deeper shade. More suggestions for lip lines in the "Reshaping" Your Features with Makeup section which follows.

"RESHAPING" YOUR FEATURES WITH MAKEUP

"What are the ideal proportions for a face?" Every now and then I am asked that question. Is there an answer? Faces don't come off an assembly line. If everyone had a classic oval, standardly spaced features, and what is known as perfect symmetry, even dedicated girl-watchers would be bored! I love the infinite variety of faces in the world. To me, there is no single "ideal" look of contemporary beauty. One needn't have eyes of a certain width, a nose of just-so length, curly hair, or a body of specific proportions. The charm of beauty lies in its *individuality*. There are as many kinds as there are women in the world, and the ones who stand out are those who have developed their own unique styles; whose looks express their personalities and interests.

Some women have good basic features but do so little to accent their looks that, like uncut gems, they pass unnoticed. Others, not so well-endowed, find the facets to accent, polish them to perfection, and turn themselves into dazzling creatures. Some of the most beautiful women I know could not pass the test of symmetrical measurement. One has a mouth too large, another a crooked smile, still another a rather long nose. Yet these women, recognizing that an irregular feature is not necessarily a flaw, have learned to use what was given to them to best advantage.

Deciding what to emphasize, what to play down is always important. If you have a really bad feature that can't be corrected, the best policy is to work on your other features until they are so perfect they draw attention away from the flaw.

Some things that can't be changed *can* be disguised. Makeup can create many optical illusions that make things seem what they aren't. Models, actresses, and photographers use color, light, and shadow to make eyes appear larger or deeper set, to create the effect of high cheekbones, to make the face appear a different shape. They have learned to lead the observer's eye and to fool it charmingly. You can create impressions of your own by following the same principles of *trompe-l'oeil.* Just keep in mind that light colors *accent,* making an area seem more prominent; dark colors *diminish,* making an area less prominent—and follow the specific directions that apply to your face.

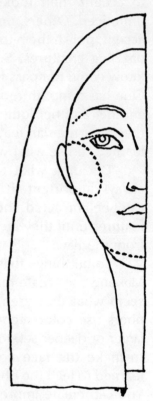

Face too long?

Apply light-toned cheek color (preferably with a glow) at the *outside* of the cheeks, starting under the outer corner of the eye. Blend the color back toward the top of the ear. At the lower part of the chin, use makeup base two tones *darker* than your normal skin-matching shade, blending it out over the jaw. Accent the outer corners of the eyes, carrying eyeliner slightly beyond end of the lid. Extend eyebrow an extra half inch toward the temple.

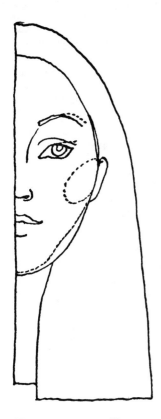

Face too round?

Don't dab color in a circle on your cheeks. Apply a tawny shade starting at the middle of the cheek, carrying it back to the temple and down almost to the jawline. Use a darker makeup base along the chin line from ear to ear to create more oval illusion. In making up the eyes, avoid a "round eye" look. Try for a longer look, with an upward tilt. Let the brows end on the upbeat too.

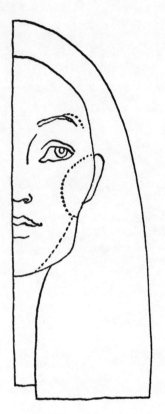

Too-square face or over-prominent jawline?

Use a darker shade of makeup base along and just under the jawbone starting below the cheekbones, blending off at the chin. Use a tawny cheek color far out on the side of the face, blending it smoothly into the darker foundation. Accent top of eyebrow, lifting the arch subtly.

Chin receding?

Use makeup base a shade *lighter* than skintone on the chin area to make it appear more prominent. Wear a touch more color high and centered on the cheeks and play up your eyes.

Nose too short or too broad?

Apply a light shade of opaque makeup base (or a light shade of the conceal/camouflage product) in a thin line right down the center of the nose, from bridge to tip. Blend lightly.

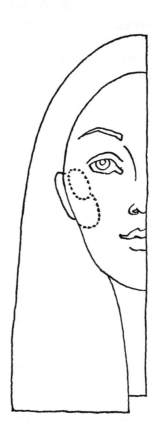

To highlight cheekbones

Use a highlight or transparent glow cheek color on the highest point of the cheekbone. In the hollow, starting at center cheek and blending off toward the ear, apply a makeup base several tones darker than natural skintone. Or use a deep or tawny blush, blending edges to avoid sharp line of demarcation.

Nose too long?

Use a darker shade of makeup base along the side of the nose, under and up onto the tip.

Double chin?

Use a darker foundation under the chin, blending edges carefully.

To "bring out" deep-set eyes

On the lid, a shade that is paler than your skintone—preferably a matte eye shadow for its opaque quality. Carry it into and just above the hollow. On the bone between lid and brow, brown or taupe shadow. A thin line of pale highlight or white shadow just under the eyebrow. Eyeliner in a very thin line on upper lid only.

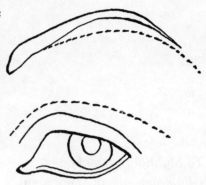

To deepen prominent eyes

On the lid—apply brown or other deep tone of matte eye shadow. On the bone between lid and brow, a lighter shade, blended right up to the brow.

To separate close-set eyes

Accent the outer corners. Start eye shadow toward the center of the lid and blend out. Begin eyeliner one half inch in from the inner corner and extend just beyond the outer end of the lid. Leave a little more separation between brows and extend them one half inch at end Blend a light shade of conceal/camouflage product between the inner corners of the eyes and bridge of the nose to give a look of added width to this area.

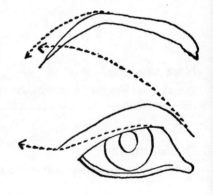

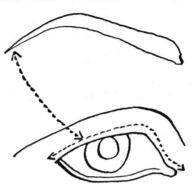

To "bring in" wide-apart eyes

Dark eye shadow at the outer edges of the lids, carried up to the brow. Start eyeliner at the inner-most corner of the eye. Do not extend it beyond the edge of the lid.

To make the eye look bigger

Between inner corners of the eye and bridge of the nose, a pale tone of conceal/camouflage makeup or light beige eye shadow. The same pale tone, at the outer corners of the eyes. A pale matte eye shadow on the lid, extended a little beyond the end of the eye. A medium shade on the bone between lid and brow, blended toward and accenting the outer corners of the eye. Eyeliner in a very thin line—starting one quarter of an inch in from inner corner—close to the lashes at first, gradually lifted a little above the lash line toward the end of the lid, extended one quarter of an inch beyond the end of lid. Give lashes two applications of mascara, using a sweeping lift (or follow with an eyelash curler) to "open up" the eyes. Frosted cheek color very high on the cheekbones to draw attention to the eye area. Eyebrows light in color. Pluck out any stray hairs from under the natural brow line; accent the top of the brow, giving the ends a slight lift.

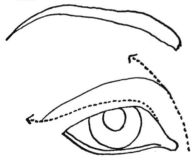

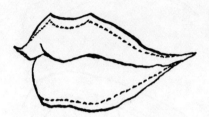

To make your mouth look smaller

When applying makeup base and powder to your face, include your lips. Draw your lipstick outline just *inside* the natural line, using a light shade. Fill in with a slightly deeper (but still light)) shade. Don't use frosted or luminous lipstick.

To make your mouth look bigger

Be sure lips have been included in application of makeup base and powder. Apply lipstick just *outside* the natural lip line, outlining in a fairly deep shade and filling in with a lighter color. Lip gloss can be added.

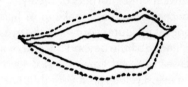

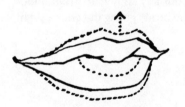

To give curves to thin lips

Foundation and powder form the base for correction. Draw a curve along lower lip, just outside the natural lip line. Outline above the bows for more fullness. Use a white highlight at center of the bottom lip and in the little valley above the lips between the center of the bows.

MAKEUP FOR A GLAMOROUS EVENING

Night—how beautifully, contrastingly different it is from day! With the setting sun, there is a change of mood—a change of look—a change of mind. The great cities of the world come alive. Champagne corks pop in Paris, Roman fashionables gather in art-hung palacios, elegant Londoners fill the glittering restaurants of Mayfair, from a terrace in San Francisco partygoers gaze at the twinkling lights of the Golden Gate. Night, anywhere, can mean counting stars from the patio, camaraderie at the country club, dinner for two by candlelight. And night, *everywhere,* is the time for a woman to drop the mantle of daytime efficiency and reveal the nocturnal side of her personality—romantic, intriguing, enigmatic perhaps, and, above all, completely womanly.

The different *you* that emerges by night is defined by your evening makeup—a very special makeup that expresses your nocturnal personality and reflects most beautifully under the starlight, moonlight, soft light, and artificial light of all the darkling hours.

Since the appearance of color is influenced by the degree and type of light, makeup that flatters under the sun can look all wrong under the moon. Even more demanding than the moon is artificial light, which tends to drain color, giving pale shades—particularly those that lean to yellow, coral, or orange—a washed-out look. As a compensation, makeup should be more vivid at nighttime. Warmer shades with undertones of pink, rose, or bronze give a soft radiance under artificial light. Luminous, frosted makeup is especially flattering. Here are a few guidelines.

Complexion makeup

Wear foundation and face powder one tone warmer than daytime shade. As an alternative, add a rosier cheek color or brush a pink blush on cheeks, lightly across forehead, on the tip of the chin. A touch of luminous highlight at the crest of the cheekbones is appealing!

Lips

Lipstick must be more vivid. Pale or whitened shades do a vanishing act. Bright pink, cherry, rose shades are good. So are burnished bronze tones. Luminous or frosted lipsticks if they are not too pale. Try a deep-rose lipstick with a paler frosted lipstick over it. Or use a non-frosted lipstick with a touch of gold or silver luminous highlight at the center of the bottom lip.

Eyes

Be imaginative in dressing the eyes for evening. Shadow can be stronger in color than for day. Use two or three shades, tone-on-tone, and luminous highlight. A line of brown, gray, or dark blue matte shadow, following the crease of the eye (the recessed area in the hollow) gives a look of depth and interest. (Omit if eyes are deep set.) Apply a thin streak of luminous highlight just under the brow. The eyeliner can be in a frosted shade of taupe, sable, blue, or green. Be sure brows are clearly defined and give the ends a slightly higher tilt.

Lashes

Stroke on two or three coats of mascara for a lush fringe to flutter as you glance provocatively over a glass of champagne—or the evening paper.

Whatever your plans, the night should be faced with appropriate makeup. If it's a gala occasion, however, it calls for an *extra* festive look. If you're adventurous, try some of the whims-of-the-moment from the latest issue of a fashion

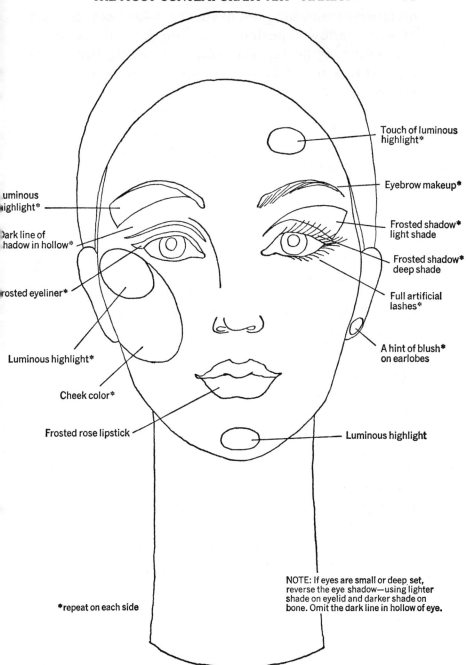

Touch of luminous highlight*

Eyebrow makeup*

Frosted shadow* light shade

Frosted shadow* deep shade

Full artificial lashes*

A hint of blush* on earlobes

Luminous highlight

Luminous highlight*

Dark line of shadow in hollow*

Frosted eyeliner*

Luminous highlight*

Cheek color*

Frosted rose lipstick

*repeat on each side

NOTE: If eyes are small or deep set, reverse the eye shadow—using lighter shade on eyelid and darker shade on bone. Omit the dark line in hollow of eye.

magazine or innovate a few of your own—an unusual shade of eye shadow, applied in an unconventional manner—eyebrows flecked with silver—an imaginative use of highlight. A bit of fantasy is fun, especially when the occasion is right!

Evening makeup can be as individual as you yourself. The preceding diagram illustrates basic evening makeup—to be adapted to your special needs, your own very personal look of glamour.

THE MANY SHADES OF LOVELY

In beauty's kaleidoscope one sees skin of every hue. The more dramatic a skintone, however, the more it may demand a special atmosphere for the display of its unique tonal quality. Here are a few of the very special skin-shade types, along with makeup recommendations to heighten their appeal . . .

THE LILY FAIR

Pale, pale—almost waxen in its beauty—this is the skin that goes beyond the fair. One of the most prized, most admired of complexions, it requires a delicate hand in makeup. Against its paleness many shades seem too obvious. All color seems intensified on this skin. Pink glares and peach looks orange. Choose, then, a pale champagne shade of liquid foundation and use it *very sparingly.* If the complexion is oily in the center area, apply the foundation to cheeks and forehead only, omitting nose and chin. Blend the edges carefully and over the entire face apply translucent face powder for a matte finish *without* the addition of color. Use a soft pink blush of color on the cheeks. Lipstick should be a clear pastel tone; avoid both vivid and whitened colors. Eye makeup must be subtle. Brow color should be soft. Eyeliner (taupe or soft blue) should be applied in a very thin line. Shadow should be in a delicate pastel shade, preferably a frosted matte. Lashes give definition but shouldn't overpower. Use light brown or ash mascara.

THE MEDITERRANEAN BRUNETTE

This is the olive complexion one might find on a Persian princess or Italian movie star. Complemented by the right colors, it takes on an exotic quality. Choose makeup foundation in a shade that has a touch of rose and, over it, apply translucent face powder. Cheek color, in a rose or tawny tone, can be used more generously on the olive skin. Keep it high on the cheekbones to draw attention to the eyes. Lipstick should be bright and clear—leaning to the vivid—with a high gloss (but not frosted). Reds and warm corals are especially attractive. The eyes must be positive magnets, strongly accented with jewel tones—clear blue, green, turquoise are lovely colors for eye shadow. Use brown eyebrow pencil and a luminous pink or beige highlight just under the brow; eyeliner in dark brown, navy green, or charcoal. Lashes should wear dark brown mascara. As a beautiful final touch, add a sunlight spot of luminous beige highlight at the crest of the cheekbones and the chin—perhaps a touch on the forehead.

THE DELICATE ORIENTAL

How exquisite is the Oriental face with its creamy, opaque complexion. The makeup foundation and powder for a perfect finish should match the skin as closely as possible, or be just a tone paler. Bisque and golden-beige shades are excellent. Follow with translucent face powder. Peach or rose blush should be applied at the crest of the cheekbone and blended back toward the ears. Almost every shade of lipstick looks attractive—especially a clear soft red or bright pink. The eyes so dominate the Oriental face that they require relatively subdued dressing. Neutral tones of eye shadow—ivory, brown, cream, white, bronze, are lovely; if color is used it should be soft—pale blue, lime, or aqua. Eyeliner should be drawn very thinly in dark brown, navy, green, or black. The brows may be defined with a charcoal shade of pencil. Black mascara on the lashes adds the lovely final touch.

THE DRAMATIC DARK

The deeper complexion tones are dramatic and provide a superb foil for exciting makeup. Whether your skintone is golden beige, warm bronze, or ebony, or if you prefer to have it referred to as black, be sure the underlying tone is matched in makeup foundation. Avoid shades with too much yellow or pink; a flat, muted tone blends in more harmoniously. Or, over the moisturizing emulsion (or pre-makeup normalizer if skin is oily), apply bronzer stick—lightly over the whole face or as an accent. Translucent face powder will give a matte, attractive finish without adding color. If the complexion is medium dark, highlight the cheekbones with amber or honey shades of blush. On the deeper complexion, use a more vivid rose tone. The eyes are usually dominant but need more emphatic framing. Brows should be brushed upward and accented with dark brown, charcoal, or black pencil. Eyeliner may be dark brown, charcoal, or black; tones of navy green or sea blue are glamorous for evening. Luminous eye shadow, colors in combination, or tone-on-tone, have special charm on the dark complexion. Try grape on the lids, shading off to heather toward the brow; add a highlight of luminous pink just under the eyebrow. Or be adventurous with shades of green—or blue—or lemon and lime. A luminous highlighter in taupe works magic on the dark complexion—touched to the crest of the cheekbone, to the sides of the eyes, a little on the chin, the brow bone, the forehead. Lashes must be lush to complete the look of beauty. Use black mascara. Bright but not frosted is the recommendation for lipstick. Select warm coral, soft red, or tawny brownish shades.

THE HAPPY MEDIUM

On every continent and in practically every country we find the woman whose coloring is neither dark nor fair and who is generally described (rather inadequately I think) as "medium." I like to call it "Happy Medium." Actually, this is the least restrictive of colorings, the one most apt to change tonality with the seasons, the one that can change its beauty personality with the flick of a lipstick and the switch of a dress. Like the chameleon, the woman who is a "Happy Medium" can take on a variety of looks. Because of her highly adaptable personal coloring, she can wear every shade in fashion's rainbow. However, to avoid being swallowed up by strong costume colors or washed out by neutrals, she must rely on makeup that plays a harmonious obbligato to every background. Depending on its accompanying setting, the face of the "Happy Medium" can take on a soft beige look, accented with warm coral lipstick, tawny cheek color, eyes shadowed with bronze or taupe or brown and highlighted with ivory tones. Or it can assume a more radiant character—skin tone brightened by foundation with a slightly rosy hue, pink or rose cheek color, lipstick with rosy-red undertones, eyes emphatically dressed in blue or green. The accent of lush lashes is important for the "Happy Medium"—brown or a brown/black mascara is attractive.

SPECIAL SITUATIONS

WHEN ANY CAMERA CLICKS

It takes less than a second for the camera to capture an image—but the result of that fleeting moment can last for years. As long as your likeness is to be preserved on film, if not for posterity at least for some degree of observation, make it as attractive as possible. From personal experience—both happy and heart-rending—I've accumulated some guidelines that you, too, may find helpful.

Plan your attire with care. Prints, dots, stripes, gimmicky accessories, detract from the subject. The camera gives a ten-pounds-heavier look, so if you're overweight, choose an outfit that's dark and slimming. A simple hair style and not too much clutter around the face is best. Most important, of course, is one's expression. Whether you're sitting for a portrait, taking a passport picture, or having your photo snapped in front of the Eiffel Tower, try to look lovely but relaxed. Try this model's trick: Concentrate all your thoughts on wishing for some wonderful treasure—take a deep breath, pretend your wish is realized, breathe out—click! That's *it!*

AT THE PHOTOGRAPHER'S STUDIO

Sitting for your portrait in black and white

The eye of the camera is more sensitive than the human eye. Let softness and subtlety be your guide! Makeup should be perfect, but lightly applied. If you pile on layer after layer, it will look masklike. If there is an obvious flaw (a pimple that appeared at the last minute) this can be retouched out of the finished picture—so don't let it ruin your day. Consider, in advance, which is your best angle—profile, three-quarter, or full face—and be sure the camera captures it.

A personal note to your portrait will diminish the austere "studio" quality. Do you have a habit of resting your beautiful long hand on the side of your face? Then do it in the picture. Do you treasure an heirloom pin? Wear it for your picture.

One personal note that *shouldn't* be added is eyeglasses. I think many people look better with them than without them—but not in formal photographs. They tend to reflect the light—and even if this is avoided they still dominate the picture. (Of course, in a casual outdoor picture, sunglasses can look great!)

In black and white pictures, color will register as degrees of gray. This is where you can make full use of the shading and highlighting techniques that seem to reshape your features. Omit rouge, unless it's very pale. Too much will come across gray, making your cheeks look flat. To highlight your cheekbones, for a sculptured look, use a lighter shade of makeup foundation on the bone and darker shade in the hollow under the cheekbone. A glow to the complexion comes across beautifully; a shiny nose doesn't! Apply translucent powder over your makeup for a matte look, then add a gleaming highlight where it does the most: the crest of the cheekbone, the chin, perhaps a touch on the forehead.

Do the best eye makeup job of your life; the eyes are the focal point of the portrait. Follow the suggestions given in "Reshaping" Your Features With Makeup that apply to *your* eyes. Use neutral tones of eye shadow—taupe, gray, brown, white—to mold the eye area. If you use colors, they must be of varying intensity—light, medium, dark—to give the degree of contrast needed for a sculptured look. Black eyebrow pencil, liner, or lashes will register much too dark. If you're a deep brunette, use dark brown, charcoal, or a brown/black blend. If your coloring is medium to fair use softer brown shades. Artificial lashes are a "must," as every professional model knows. Find the style that is best for you. Generally, a fine, upswept style is better than a heavy lash for photography.

Lips should be pretty and curvy, but they shouldn't steal the scene. A medium pastel (or soft red on darker subject) is advisable. If lips need more shape, outline them in a deeper tone and fill in with a paler shade, but blend the colors together carefully where they meet. Use a glossy lipstick, or a gloss stick over regular lipstick, for a shiny look.

Sitting for your portrait in color

Here the camera's eye is supersensitive! It registers color more vividly than the eye does, so aim for an understated makeup. Even if vivid tones are flattering to you for general use, forego them for this occasion. Follow the rules for reshaping features, as they apply to your face, but choose tones with less contrast than those used for black and white photography. Use skin-matching makeup foundation over your entire face; for shading and highlighting choose shades only one tone lighter or deeper. A touch of blush on the cheeks is attractive; peach or a light tawny tone is good. Do beautiful things with your eyes, using shades that are muted and matte. Avoid black liner, pencil, lashes—use charcoal or soft brown instead. A beige luminous highlight just under the brow, on the chin, at the crest of the brow, is attractive. Don't let your lips upstage your eyes; a soft pastel or light tawny tone of lipstick will give enough definition.

Sitting for an amateur photographer

All the foregoing hints apply—but watch those lights! A professional photographer knows how to avoid unflattering shadows. If your friend doesn't, don't sit until he learns. Overhead lights cause shadows around the eyes and cheeks, make the nose and forehead stand out. Lighting from below points up any flaws in the contour. Lighting from the sides and from behind the face is more flattering.

OR MAYBE INSTAMATIC?

It's casual, informal, sometimes candid. You're not going to make elaborate preparations, but you don't want to wince when the snapshots are passed around. If a camera is going along on the excursion, don't wear the dress with horizontal stripes that day. Or the geometric print. Or a belt that cuts your figure in half. And do give a little extra attention to your makeup—particularly the eyes, which need definition.

Watch your posture; be sure your back is straight, chest high, and chin lifted slightly to chase shadows from the face.

IF YOU'RE ON TV

When television was born, it immediately killed that old *réchauffé* "the camera does not lie." Lie it did. And distort. Even worse, it was sometimes too honest!

During its inception, one of my special projects was to create makeup for this new medium. I recall pre-telecast sessions with some of the great stars of Broadway, Hollywood, and radio, who approached the "monster" with quaking fear.

One night a famous actress who was about to make her TV debut tried to bolt at the zero hour. She was rushing for the door when I called out to her that a covey of fans were waiting outside for her autograph—and if they saw her in her TV makeup she was doomed! I'm not sure if there was actually a group at the other side of the door, but I *do* know that the stylized TV makeup of those early days would have been grotesque in street light, even on her lovely face! Yes, she did go through with the show and projected a glamorous image on all her fans' TV screens!

Television has made tremendous strides. The camera is no longer feared, and television makeup has become a special art. In large studios, professional makeup artists assist performers and celebrity guests. However, should it happen that you'll be facing TV cameras without such expert help, keep these tips in mind:

FOUNDATION

Use an opaque makeup base for flawless coverage. Three shades are needed:

1. Basic foundation shade—closest to your natural skintone
2. Highlight foundation shade—2 or 3 tones lighter
3. Toner foundation shade—3 or 4 tones darker

First, smooth basic foundation shade over the face, ears, neck, décolletage, entire exposed area. Next, apply the highlight shade on ridges from corners of nose to mouth, on areas of the face to be "brought forward"—receding chin, too-hollow cheeks, for example. Apply the darker shade over areas to be receded—heavy jowls, double chin, in the cheek hollows if a more sculptured look is desired. Blend all edges carefully to avoid sharp demarcation between tones.

Be sure to avoid very pale basic foundation shade as it will give a ghostly look, or intense tone which may register too harshly. Soft beige and rose or peach tones—or bronze for dark skin—are excellent basic foundation shades.

FACE POWDER

Translucent face powder will give a matte finish over all foundation shades and will not diminish the effect of shading and highlighting.

EYE MAKEUP

Very dark shades of eyebrow makeup or eyeliner look too harsh on the TV screen. Dark brunettes will find dark brown preferable to black. Medium or fair subjects should wear light brown, taupe, or charcoal.

Use several shades of eye shadow for "contouring" the eye area. Lighter shades will make an area seem more prominent; darker shades will tend to recede.

Subtle tones of pale blue, aqua, lime or heather are good on the lid, with deeper tones on the brow bone for a feeling of depth.

Emphasize the lashes with mascara or use artificial lashes.

CHEEKS

Concentrate on contouring with color—a soft blush on the

cheekbone, a darker tone in the hollow. Blend all edges carefully. Avoid too much color or too deep a tone. When in doubt, "less" is preferable to "more."

LIPSTICK
The camera transmits red more vividly than it appears to the naked eye. Avoid darker tones. Warm coral tones, golden or beige tones are recommended, with a slightly darker shade outlining the lips. If frosted lipstick is used, choose a medium shade, as reflection will make a light shade register too pale.

WHEN YOU'RE A GOOD SPORT

Women who enjoy sports have asked me from time to time if it isn't better to leave off face makeup ("so that my skin can breathe") while they're active at play. The answer is no. With all outdoor sports, your skin is exposed to the potentially damaging rays of the sun (whatever the season), to wind, often to dust, and in winter to intense cold. All these factors dry, coarsen, and in one way or another hurt the skin. Whatever you can put between your skin and the elements, including makeup, is to your skin's advantage.

Before going out, use a rich moisturizer and pat eye cream around the eyes. After the cream has been completely absorbed, apply a sunscreen product. You will be able to apply makeup smoothly over a greaseless type. Be sure to use plenty of lipstick. Lip tissue is especially delicate and vulnerable. Use a creamy or moisturizing eye shadow, for extra protection of the lids.

Whatever your sport, carry a sunscreen product and eye cream in your bag or keep extras at your club locker so that you may reapply frequently.

Reflected light from sand, water, or snow can be especially damaging. Skiers and other winter-sports lovers should be aware that the intensity of sunlight is 20 percent greater at 5,000 feet above sea level and increases with altitude. Skip face makeup if you like, and keep slathering your face with a heavy-duty sunscreen product. Then by all means use a ski mask. You can show your prettiest face, and an undamaged one, in perfect makeup après ski!

Joggers (and other good sports) who perspire heavily are apt to lose a lot of moisture from their skin. Give your skin *extra* moisturizing care: use moisturizer on your face before and after jogging and also routinely under makeup and at bedtime. Use a moisturizing body lotion after showering. "Moisturize" from the inside, too, by drinking plenty of water.

WHEN THE SEASON CHANGES

Your clothes change, too! The traditional pattern was darker colors for winter, paler ones for spring, brighter shades for summer, richer for fall. Even if you don't follow that pattern, you probably enjoy the refreshing change of colors from season to season. As your fashions change, analyze your makeup—and adjust for harmony.

A change of season generally means a change of skin tone. If you tan in summer, your face makeup must "tan" with you and "fade" as you lose your tan later. To adjust your foundation, you'll need your basic shade and a darker one. As your skin deepens in color, blend in the palm of your hand a touch of the darker shade with the basic shade. Try a bit on the jawline to test for color. When you've got the right shade, smooth all over your face.

With a tan, wear a coral or warm, tawny tone of lipstick; soft green, turquoise, or brown tones of eye shadow. Even if you don't purposely cultivate a tan, your skin may darken somewhat from the exposure it gets in everyday comings and goings. Check your makeup to be sure it's right for the season.

At season's end, a fading tan can give a dull and even a sallow look. Add an extra touch of blush high on the cheekbones—apply blush ever so lightly on the temples or just around the hairline at the forehead. If you're young and pert, try a very light brushing of tawny blush from the top of the cheekbones right across the bridge of the nose (the freckle band). Use a vivid lipstick and, if brows have been bleached by the sun, pencil them for more definition.

WHEN YOU'RE TRAVELING

Going to another part of the world may mean a change of season for your face. However, rather than the gradual change that occurs at home, there can be the shock of sudden change within a few hours. Apart from temperature and climate change, your skin will be affected by change of diet and sometimes by the difference in the water it's washed with.

I always pack my skin care and makeup products with as much care as I do my clothes for a trip of any distance. Moisturizers are especially important. Skin tends to dry, in most cases, so take along a smoothing body lotion. You'll want to massage your feet with it, too, after a long day of sightseeing.

Plastic containers with good tight caps are your best bet, as they're lightweight and will hold just the amount you need for your trip. Be sure to label them carefully. You'd be surprised how easy it is to forget which is which!

One of the important things to take on a vacation trip is a facial mask. Generally there is a quiet hour at the end of the afternoon when you're resting before preparing for dinner. It's an hour you rarely find at home, so luxuriate—enjoy relaxing, and spend at least twenty minutes of it with a refreshing mask on your face!

5
The All of You

Can you imagine anything more wonderful than the female body? So intricate and yet so precise in its working, so delicate yet resilient, so sensitive yet strong—and so beautiful to behold! The form that has inspired sculptors, painters, poets, and just plain mortals should be valued as your greatest treasure, which, in fact, it is. Call it a mechanical marvel or an aesthetic delight—your body is *you.* It's the you that ticks. It's the you that moves with the grace of a woodland creature or the leaden weight of Tugboat Annie. It's the you that is looked over with admiration—or overlooked.

A beautiful body means many things to a woman. It is a clear manifestation of her femininity. As the instrument of her sexuality, it spells desirability to her man. It pleases all eyes that focus on her. It bespeaks her discipline, her values, her life-style. The truly beautiful body radiates good health. The you that shows on the outside is the product of constant activity inside. The words "blood circulation, digestive system, glandular secretions, respiratory action" are neither lyrical nor glamorous—yet these body works are the *real* glamour producers. A clear, radiant complexion, eyes that sparkle, shining hair, strong nails, a trim figure, a spring in the step, energy to spare—and *joie de vivre* that a million dollars couldn't buy. All these are gifts of good physical condition. If you want to enjoy them now, and if you have a beautiful future in mind, you must decide to give your body the good attention it deserves.

A Medical Check-Up
Think of it as a once-a-year favor you do for yourself. Your doctor can tell you whether you're on the right track for happy, healthy living and can detect any minor problem before it becomes major.

An Eye Examination
Whether or not you wear glasses now, make a visit to an eye doctor a yearly "must." What possession is more precious than your eyes?

Regular Dental Checkups
Visit your dentist at least twice a year. It's your best way of keeping small dental problems from turning into big ones—and keeping your winning smile!

The Right Food
What you eat and drink determines how you look, how you feel, what you are. Nutrition is so closely related to your attractiveness that a complete section on "Food for Beauty" follows.

Exercise
It's great for body tone, for circulation, for so many things that go on inside your body. There's a complete section on exercise a few pages on. If you have the least thought of skipping it, then it's *especially* for you!

Beauty Sleep
Among your most important hours are the eight you

reserve for your body to rest, rejuvenate itself, and awaken to a lovelier day. The quality of your sleep is as important as the quantity. Unless you're one of the fortunates beloved by Morpheus, you may want to consider some slumber inducers: tension-relieving exercise half an hour before bed, a glass of warm milk, a tepid bath, a splash of light cologne, pleasant music, and a book of poetry before you turn out the light. Fundamental to sound sleep and to a strong spine, of course, is a good firm mattress.

Leisure Pleasure

We know what happened to Jack's personality rating because of "all work." It wasn't good for his body either. We hear too often of chronic illness due to stress. Nor is "all play" the answer, even for the rare few who have the choice. Most human beings thrive on a balance of both work and relaxation. And relaxation doesn't mean collapse; it means change. One whose day is filled with mental effort and tension without great physical activity will find release in an after-hours game of tennis, ice skating, or dancing (even partnerless and in her own room if need be). One whose daytime activities involve considerable physical exertion may experience a refreshing change of pace by attending a concert or class, reading an absorbing book, or in stimulating conversation with friends. Every life should include several interests; things to which one is deeply committed or keenly enjoys. Only when there is a balance of rewarding pursuit do the body and mind blend to create a healthy, happy "All of You."

HOW DO YOU SHAPE UP?

Now—step right up to a full-length mirror and take a long, honest, up-and-down look. That's *you*—all of you. I've spoken about rules to follow for a lovely complexion and how to dress it in the most enhancing makeup. Later, we'll discuss hair—which you can learn to handle yourself or put in the hands of an expert hair stylist. But what about you from the neck down? Is your body slim, firm, lithe, and lovely? Or is it in need of alteration? You wouldn't plan a trip without being sure of your starting point and your destination and without a clear road map. And you'll reach your goal of a good figure more easily if you know, in inches and pounds, where your figure stands right now and where you want it to be.

For this important self-analysis, find a completely private time when you can stand nude, or in your scanties, before a full-length mirror. First let your eyes note any obvious disproportion. Now do some finger-tip checking. Squeeze the flesh around your waist, your thighs, upper arms, neck. Is it all firm tissue? Or is there too much looseness, the beginning of flabbiness? Next, check the inches with a tape measure:

Neck	under the chin
Bust	fullest circumference
Diaphragm	2″ below the bust
Waist	narrowest part
Hips	at the hipbone
Thighs	fullest part
Calf	fullest part
Ankle	at the bone
Arms	just under the armpit

Write the measurements on an index card, with the date, leaving space for entering comparative statistics at monthly intervals. Weigh yourself and jot that figure down also. Do you need to lose weight? How much? Or do you need to gain? Make a note of the areas that need firming or reproportioning. Are the upper arms a little flabby? The thighs too heavy? Is the stomach hard and flat? How is your posture? Does your head sit straight on your spine or does it droop? Is your derrière tucked under, your chest held high?

Recommended weights are listed below. Frame is determined by your bone structure. If you have small wrists, ankles, hands, and neck, yours is a small frame. If you have wide shoulders, a broad pelvis, large wrists, you have a large frame. Most people fit into a "medium" classification. Muscle structure is also a factor to consider. A well-toned body with firm, "well-packed" flesh may weigh at the top of the range shown, but appear pounds thinner.

WHAT SHOULD YOU WEIGH?

Height	Small Frame	Medium Frame	Large Frame
5'0"	95–100	100–105	108–112
5'1"	95–100	105–110	110–115
5'2"	100–105	107–112	115–120
5'3"	105–112	112–115	118–125
5'4"	108–115	115–120	120–130
5'5"	112–120	118–125	125–135
5'6"	115–122	123–130	128–138
5'7"	120–125	125–135	130–140
5'8"	122–130	127–137	140–150

Statistic noting at regular intervals is recommended for every woman. If your figure is perfect, the record will serve as your control; you'll be sure, as time goes by, that you are retaining your ideal proportions. If your figure needs improvement, you have a starting point from which to show progress and as you record it month by month you'll be encouraged to see how far you have moved in the right direction.

Your figure is shaped by diet, exercise, and posture. All must take important roles in your design for living—whether your aim is finding a new figure or retaining the perfect one you have.

FOOD FOR BEAUTY

Munch. Crunch. Sip. How many bites and swallows did you take today? Was it just food—or food for beauty?

What you eat and drink does far more than dispel hunger and slake thirst. It fuels your body to keep the whole intricate mechanism working. It smooths—or bumps—your complexion. It brightens—or dulls—your eyes. It builds firm tissue—or flab. It helps you feel joyfully alive—or sluggishly existent.

We've all heard the plump lady coaxing the slim lady to have another pastry, with the assurance "With *your* figure you can eat anything!" Probably the slim lady will decline (she loves wearing size 8) and as for eating "anything" she *mustn't.* Not if she wants to hold onto her good health as well as her good looks.

I wish all women could find the salad bowl as tempting as the pastry tray. And I would love to see women approach a greengrocer's display with as much excitement as they do a cosmetic counter. Packed into those curly green leaves, behind that citrus peel, in all those wares of Nature, are the most effective beauty aids of all. I'm not advocating that you become a food fanatic or that you spend hours browsing in the health food shop. Not unless it gives you special pleasure. Most nutritionists agree that you needn't go to extremes. Unless your doctor has recommended a special diel for specific reasons, just follow the simple, proven way.

Let's consider basic principles of nutrition that apply to everyone.

VITAMINS AND MINERALS—
Everybody's food friends!

Since these essentials are scattered in many foods, a well-varied diet provides the best insurance of getting your quota. Vitamin A fights infection, repairs tissue, does sparkling things for eyes. It's in liver, carrots, spinach, cantaloupe. B complex helps the body utilize nutrients and keeps glands on the go. Find the B's in wheat germ, yogurt, milk, bananas, chicken. Vitamin C makes building blocks for connective tissue, helps form red blood cells, puts strength in teeth and gums. It's in citrus fruits, strawberries, broccoli, sprouts. The sunshine one, D, is in eggs, milk, tuna fish. Since vitamins can be dissipated or even destroyed by overcooking, to enjoy them at their most potent, eat some raw fruits and vegetables every day. And try serving slightly undercooked vegetables. They're crisply flavorful and more vitamin-filled. The good foods that deliver vitamins also provide the minerals essential for good health and good looks. Iron is in liver, wheat germ, spinach. Calcium is in milk, broccoli, cottage cheese. Phosphorus is in fish and poultry; potassium in leafy green vegetables. Salt (sodium) is a mineral to shun, or at least to use very sparingly, as too much can contribute to serious bodily ills—starting with hypertension.

PROTEIN—The hero of our food story!

This great do-gooder works together with the vitamins and minerals in your diet to form blood, bone, tissue; to regulate the body's operation; to keep the flesh firm and the body vital. The greatest concentrations of protein are found in lean meat, fish, and poultry. It's also present in many other foods in varying proportions. Skim milk, soybeans, lentils, cheese, eggs, are good sources—though these also contain some carbohydrates and fats.

CARBOHYDRATES—Moderation is the watchword.

Carbohydrates provide important nutrients for growing children and young people under twenty. After that, in moderation, they serve a vital metabolic purpose. Carbohydrates deliver quick energy, satisfy hunger, and chase fatigue. People engaged in strenuous physical labor need and use more carbohydrates than those who lead more sedentary lives. A lumberjack can polish off a stack of pancakes; a secretary shouldn't. An intake of more carbohydrates than your body can use contributes to flabby flesh (versus protein's firm production), overweight, and eventually a depletion of energy. Some carbohydrates, in most advantageous form, are found in vegetables and fruits. Heaviest concentrations are in bread, flour, cakes, potatoes, pasta, rice, cereals.

SUGARS—Too sweet to be true.

Sugars are a form of carbohydrate, and like some cloying people, they can be very sticky. Refined sugar comes from sugar cane (in some countries from the sugar beet). However, almost all foods contain a small measure of sugar. The amount needed by the normal body, for correct sugar-level balance, is provided by staple foods such as vegetables, breads, some meats, and especially fruits. Most people do not require any visible sugar, such as the granulated kind. Refined sugar has no food value—just calories. Hard candies, chocolates, soft drinks, all sugar-laden, are bad for the teeth, the figure—and often for the complexion too. If you crave something sweet, reach for a piece of fruit. It's a natural source of sugar, but has vitamins and minerals too. On cereals or desserts that need sweetening, use honey as a substitute—it has many good food qualities and is one of the most wholesome sugar sources.

FATS—Too often villainous!

The body needs a certain amount of fat, true—for body heat, for lubrication of the skin and hair, for essential metabolism. The required amount is generally derived from the natural fat content of dairy products, meats, and other staples. The watchword is *restraint.* Too much fat wreaks havoc on the digestive and vascular systems, contributes to an overoily complexion and enlarged pores. Whether you're thin, plump, or just right—avoid, whenever you can, fried foods, rich pastries, fat-filled dressings. Go easy on foods such as bacon, cream, mayonnaise, nuts, olives, butter. Trim visible fat from meats. A light vegetable- or seed-derived oil, for cooking or salads, is preferable to heavier oils, lard, etc.—but even that must be used in moderation.

SIP FOR BEAUTY

WATER—ESPECIALLY! Pindar told the ancient Greeks "Water is best." And it still is. It has a cleansing, refreshing value for the inside as well as the outside of the body. For a clear complexion and a host of other advantages, drink eight glasses daily—between, never with, meals. If the tap water in your area is not inspiring, buy bottled spring water. Drink it from finest crystal, a champagne glass if you wish. However you do it, learn to appreciate water for the vital beauty maker it is.

COFFEE AND TEA. These are comforting pick-me-ups. Some people have greater tolerance than others for the caffein and tannic acid they contain. Just don't overdo on these stimulants because shaky nerves, fitful sleep, muddy-looking skin can result. Caffein-free coffee is a good alternative, especially for the between-meals cup or that late-at-night one. Try to savor the true flavor of coffee without sugar and cream, or cultivate a taste for clear tea served only with lemon. At the time I lived in London, I was trying to cut down on calories. My first step was to eliminate sugar from tea and coffee. Although my taste buds felt terribly deprived at first, I soon came to realize that either beverage is more refreshing without the additive. What's more, I now *prefer* unsweetened coffee and tea—another example of taste bud "retraining"!

ALCOHOLIC BEVERAGES. Liquor can be delightful in moderation. A drink or two before dinner is pleasantly relaxing, and many a party has owed its success to sparkles of wit lit by the sociable cocktail. Most doctors agree that a controlled amount of liquor won't hurt. What *does* hurt is excess. A puffy look, blotchiness, and other unattractive external signs merely hint at what's happening to the liver and other organs. At a recent party, I heard a man comment, "Nothing turns me off quicker than a woman who's had too much to drink." This man was no teetotaler himself, but how right he was. Every effort a woman may have made to look and be attractive is lost when that "one drink too many" results in slackened expression, twisted words, inane actions.

FRUIT JUICES (UNSWEETENED) AND VEGETABLE JUICES. These are my between-meal favorites for energy and to dispel the urge to nibble. Along with a flavorful pick-up they deliver vitamins and minerals. Use them instead of soft drinks. There are many delectable juices ready-made at your food store, or you can concoct your own combinations for interesting health cocktails. If you're counting calories, enjoy the juice of half a lemon in a glass of water for between-meals refreshment.

SHEDDING POUNDS

If weight is a serious problem—see your doctor. If you are more than ten pounds above the normal for your height, or if excess pounds cling despite a regulated diet—get professional attention. Major weight loss calls for heroic measures to be prescribed and guided by your physician. And, of course, only he can diagnose any metabolic or other physical factor that may contribute to the problem.

However, the majority of overweight people are not actually obese—just too "well-padded" for attractive appearance and for their own well-being. In the overwhelming majority of cases, this excess weight is due to one simple fault: Taking in more calories in food than are expended in energy.

The pounds creep on slowly. If you don't weigh and record regularly, you may not be aware of that rounder waistline until your favorite dress hugs too tightly. Or you may not notice the difference in your thighs until, after a covered-up winter, they are unconcealable that first day at the beach. Very often, the change is so gradual that a woman cherishes the illusion of normal proportions when in reality she is well on her way to dumpling plumpness!

You may not be eating more than you did previously—or more than your skinny sister—but obviously you are eating incorrectly for *you*. In many cases the overweight body is actually *under*-nourished in vital proteins and health-giving nutrients, while it is being too generously fed with foods it doesn't need. Perhaps there are too many fats and carbohydrates in your diet—too many cups of coffee with sugar and cream—perhaps you "splurge" occasionally by choosing the richest thing on the menu—perhaps, when you feel the grip of frustration, you console yourself with a fattening treat. In all probability you are less physically active than you were before. Obviously, you are not using up all the caloric fuel you are taking in.

Your biggest and most difficult hurdle may be your own mental attitude. Spending half an hour in serious contemplation could lead to the beginning of your new figure—and your new life. Be completely honest with yourself. Have you gained weight out of sheer indifference or loneliness, because of tension or lack of willpower? Whatever the reason, consider the consequences. I have never heard of a problem solved by overweight, but I do know of many happy solutions brought about by weight loss! Aside from your personal life: the admiration of your friends, children, husband, or that still-to-be-encountered man; the approval of your business associates; the joy of wearing clothes with fashionable flair; consider your actual physical life. It will be longer and healthier with normal weight. Excess pounds burden the body; eventually the blood pressure and heart are affected. Obesity can have dire effects that we don't like to think about—but DO think about them. No matter how tempting the roll and butter, the second helping, the pastry, is it worth it? Take time to firm up your resolve. If others can discipline themselves, so can you. You can revise your eating habits. You can train your taste buds to enjoy the things that are good for you and to reject your food "enemies." You can adjust your design for living.

After making up your mind firmly and unequivocally that you *will* acquire an attractive new figure—and the many joys that come with it—you are ready to form your definite plan. Only by balancing your diet—adjusting your caloric intake to your energy output—can you lose pounds. Of course, your diet must be teamed with a program of exercise, to keep your body firm and to redistribute weight for more pleasing proportions.

Over the years, I have worked with many doctors in

planning figure-control programs—and have discussed weight problems with untold numbers of women. Many of the women who came to Helena Rubinstein Body Salons were motivated by a crisis in their lives. Often it was a wandering husband, sometimes a lost lover, or a much-wanted job that didn't materialize. These women were filled with unhappiness and with pleas of, "Help me. I'll do anything." Yet, many expected a magic formula, some voodoo to produce maximum change with minimum effort. It doesn't work that way. Overweight is generally the result of overindulgence. Losing it takes sacrifice, self-control, and maybe a few hunger pangs. It also takes patience. Excess weight, particularly if it has been on the body for some time, can't be shed too quickly. Just consider how long it took to gain it!

From study, observation, and many case histories, I am convinced that "instant off" diets reduce a woman's resolve more than her figure. Appetite-depressant pills, especially when taken without qualified medical guidance, can bring undesirable side effects. Drastic "starvation" diets, or fad diets that disrupt normal eating patterns often work short-range.

At times I have prescribed a "crash" diet when it meant salvation for an actress who had to lose ten or fifteen pounds before the cameras were to start rolling. However, "quick" is not easy and it's not the answer for *you*—unless that last telephone call was from a producer! And for good reason. Most fad diets rigidly limit the choice of foods and, consequently, fail to deliver all the essential nutrients the body needs. At the end of the diet period (hopefully short) the dieter may experience such craving that she goes overboard for every food in sight. Or she may congratulate herself on her remarkable loss of weight but—not having established new lifetime eating patterns—will revert to her former food habits and her former weight. Do you know the woman whose "stop and go" crash dieting caused her husband such suffering (women's nervous outbursts are hard to take) that he protested his preference for her "rounded" look, claimed, "there's more of you to love" (a banality she enjoyed believing), and was last seen ogling the prettiest bikini wearer at the club? I know her—a few of her, in fact!

Rather than a short-cut, short-range, and ultimately short-change plan, adopt one that will assure permanent improvement—a design for living that brings buoyant health, energy, and zest along with a trim silhouette.

To begin your plan—and forever after—you must observe the Ten Commandments of Slimming:

THE TEN COMMANDMENTS OF SLIMMING

1. Eat three meals daily, at regular hours. Skipping breakfast or lunch can hurt your health, your disposition, your resolve.
2. Keep meals high in nutrients, low in calories. Concentrate on protein foods, vegetables, and fruit. Keep starches and fats to an absolute minimum. And never a second helping!
3. Don't nibble between meals. If you feel an irresistible urge for food, chew celery, raw carrot, or have a glass of water or tomato juice.
4. Drink eight glasses of water daily *between* meals.

Don't drink water or other beverages with meals. Wait half an hour after finishing a meal.

5. Eat slowly. Chew your food thoroughly.
6. Use very little salt in cooking. Don't add salt at the table.
7. Trim any visible fat from meat before cooking. Broil, bake, braise, or boil any cooked food. Avoid fried foods
8. If you "taste" while you're cooking, you can consume a considerable number of calories before the food even gets to the table. Measure your ingredients so that sampling won't be necessary. And if you fail to resist, you must deduct from your dinner plate the amount you sampled in the kitchen.
9. Plan beautiful meals. Set your table or tray with attractive dishes. Place flowers or a pretty centerpiece on the table. Arrange the food for eye appeal. Splurge on design, not calories.
10. Spend your energy. Stored-up calories, as we know, turn to fat. Use them wisely in daily exercise, outdoors and in. Walk, don't ride. Dance, don't dawdle. Find an activity that is enjoyable, absorbing, available, and pursue it with a passion.

And, please, when you're dieting don't talk about it. The subject is between you and your willpower. It bores everyone else. At a dinner party, take just the smallest portion on your plate. Second helpings or forbidden foods can be declined politely but firmly. You needn't give a reason. Your slimmer, lovelier figure wll speak *for* you later on!

AND NOW FOR YOUR THREE-STEP REDUCING PLAN . . .

Setting a new pattern isn't easy. To help women over that difficult "hump," the adjustment to new eating habits, I devised my Three-step Reducing Diet, which has carved some sylphlike figures from former chubbies on both sides of the Atlantic.

STEP ONE

Your first week to a slim figure. Remind yourself daily of the beautiful future in store. Visualize yourself in a smaller size dress (or bathing suit). This week you will eliminate sugar and cream from coffee or tea; add skim milk if you must. Cut out all pastries, candies, bread. Eat more leafy green vegetables and raw fruit. Drink more water—six to eight glasses daily between meals. Start exercising ten minutes daily. That's all—your first week is a breeze!

STEP TWO

Second week and you're feeling brighter, more energetic already! This week continue the new habits of Step One (and, of course, the Slimming Laws) and add just a bit more effort. Replace any whole milk—in glass, cereal, or cooking—with skim milk. Cut out gravies and sauces. For dessert, take only fruit, cheese and crackers, or gelatin, *all in small quantities*. Eat more raw vegetables: carrots, celery, salads, tomatoes. Add a daily walk of at least one mile and increase your calisthenic schedule to fifteen minutes daily. Do a joyful dance around your room now and then.

STEP THREE

Notice something different? Your willpower is showing. Now you're ready for serious diet planning, based on calorie counting with careful balance of nutrients. How many calories do you need? The average woman requires about 15 daily for each pound of her body weight. Since calories represent energy units, the greater your energy output, the more calories your body uses. A physically active woman may need 20 per pound. To shed weight, however, you must reduce your calories to 500 fewer per day than the average requirement for your weight. At that rate, you can shed one pound a week—which is realistic and less shattering to the body than rapid loss. Step Three marks the start of your calorie-counted diet. Here is a week's menu, based on 1,400 calories daily, which is filled with nutriment, satisfying, and effective. Use it as a guide, making adjustments only within the same calorie count. If you get hungry between meals, save your lunchtime dessert until 3:30—or take your dinnertime bouillon at 4:00.

After the first week of Step Three, if you've faithfully followed the Ten Commandments and the Step Three Diet I menu, you deserve a treat. The Step Three Diet II menu shows simple ways to modify the week's menu, with the addition of only 150 to 200 calories daily. Both physical activity and cold weather encourage the body to burn up calories more quickly. When either situation applies, go ahead—enjoy an extra 200 calories a day!

Does alcohol fit into the Three-Step Diet? If that question is on your mind, remember that alcoholic beverages are high in calories, but lacking in nutrition. If you can substitute mineral water with a twist of lemon for your customary drink, so much the better. If not, limit yourself to one drink a day. Dry white wine is your best choice, as it has fewer calories than hard liquor. If you take scotch, bourbon, vodka, or gin, have it with water or soda—no sweetened mixer. Absolutely no cordials, sweet wines, beer, Manhattans, Daiquiris, or other calorie-heavy cocktails!

Step Three continues until you have attained ideal weight. Then you may allow yourself a few more calories, but do continue to control your eating habits. Following a nutritious maintenance diet will be easier if you will be adventurous in finding low-calorie, high-protein recipes to add spice to your meals. There are many sources and endless possibilities.

CALORIES DAILY—APPROX. 1,400

	MONDAY	TUESDAY	WEDNESDAY	THURSDAY	FRIDAY	SATURDAY	SUNDAY
BREAKFAST	½ grapefruit 1 poached egg 1 slice toast Coffee or tea*	1 whole orange Cereal with skim milk Coffee or tea*	½ grapefruit 1 soft-boiled egg 1 slice toast Coffee or tea*	1 whole orange Shredded Wheat with skim milk Coffee or tea*	½ grapefruit 1 poached egg 1 slice toast Coffee or tea*	1 whole orange Cereal with skim milk Coffee or tea*	½ grapefruit 1 soft-boiled egg 1 slice toast Coffee or tea*
LUNCH	Vegetable salad with cottage cheese 1 slice pumpernickel bread 1 piece fresh fruit	Lean hamburger Small tomato and lettuce salad 1 slice whole wheat bread	Tomato aspic in lettuce 1 Rye Krisp or 2 graham crackers 2 sticks celery 1 raw carrot	Salad bowl of grated raw vegetables (lemon juice) ½ cup cottage cheese 1 Rye Krisp or 2 graham crackers	½ cantaloupe filled with cottage cheese 1 slice pumpernickel bread	Fresh fruit salad 1 slice toast 1 yogurt	Tomato juice 1 cup clam chowder 1 Rye Krisp or 2 graham crackers
DINNER	1 cup clear soup Roast beef (no fat) Small baked potato Lettuce and tomato salad with lemon juice Fruit compote (unsweetened)	1 cup clear soup Broiled fish Yellow squash Spinach ¼ cantaloupe	Small green salad—½ tbsp. dressing or lemon only Calves liver Green beans Small boiled potato 1 piece fresh fruit	1 cup clear soup Small lean steak Asparagus (6 spears) 1 slice Melba toast Small wedge honeydew melon	Lettuce and cucumber salad Broiled lamb chop Cauliflower 1 small boiled potato 1 cup unsweetened applesauce	1 cup clear soup Broiled fish Peas Carrots ½ cup rice 1 fresh peach or 3 apricots	Celery and raw carrot sticks Broiled chicken Asparagus (4 spears) 1 small baked potato 1 small piece of cheddar cheese/2 crackers

*No cream or sugar.
Limit all foods to one modest helping. (Example—1 cup of any vegetable shown.) A glass of skim milk or 1 plain fat-free yogurt may be taken before bed each night.

STEP THREE DIET II

	MONDAY	TUESDAY	WEDNESDAY	THURSDAY	FRIDAY	SATURDAY	SUNDAY
BREAKFAST	Same as Diet I Unsweetened grapefruit juice may be substituted for fresh fruit if desired.	Same as Diet I	Same as Diet I Add mid-morning or mid-afternoon 1 glass skim milk	Same as Diet I	Same as Diet I	Same as Diet I	Turn breakfast into brunch today. ½ grapefruit 1 scrambled egg flavored with a dash of curry 1 toasted English muffin, *lightly* spread with margarine — mid-afternoon: glass of skim milk
LUNCH	Fresh Fruit Plate (no banana) with ½ cup of cottage cheese. 1 slice pumpernickel bread mid-afternoon: 1 glass skim milk	Same as Diet I	3 oz. tuna fish (water-packed), flavored with lemon 2 Rye Krisp or 1 piece of whole wheat bread 2 sticks of celery	Same as Diet I	Smoked or canned salmon (3 oz.) 1 pc. whole wheat bread 2 celery sticks	Fresh vegetable salad 1 pc. whole wheat bread 1 small piece of Swiss cheese	

	MONDAY	TUESDAY	WEDNESDAY	THURSDAY	FRIDAY	SATURDAY	SUNDAY
DINNER	3-4 raw oysters or 4 oz. shrimp, flavored with lemon 2 plain crackers Balance of dinner same as in Diet I.	Filet of Sole (flounder or fluke) poached in white wine with 4 grapes ½ cup brown rice broccoli ¼ cantaloupe spinach	Same as Diet I For dessert substitute ½ grapefruit baked with 1 tsp honey	Baked Chicken with orange & lemon slices ½ cup spaghetti (no sauce) 5 small slices zucchini, lightly steamed watercress salad baked apple (no sugar, no cream)	Lean broiled steak or roast beef spinach 1 ear of corn, with 1 tsp margarine 1 small banana sliced in skim milk	Same as Diet I	Vegetable or tomato juice Roast chicken 1 small baked potato Brussels sprouts strawberries in wine (no sugar)

Your Three-step Diet must be combined with *daily exercise.* Only a calorie-controlled diet will help you to lose pounds, but exercise will act to firm the body and to distribute your weight for better proportions. Your scale will show the results of your diet; your tape measure the advantage of exercise.

MAINTAINING IDEAL WEIGHT

Once you've reached your ideal weight, vow to hold it there. Doing so may call for your strongest determination and a new design for living, but the rewards are many. The greatest may be that wonderful feeling of confidence that springs from *knowing* your figure is lean, lithe, and attractive. There's pleasure, too, in reaching for a favorite dress from the past and finding it still looks great; in not having to invest in a new wardrobe (or expensive alterations) because of weight fluctuation.

Even more important than these immediate satisfactions—by holding your weight at the same point you'll be healthier and younger looking all your life. Cycles of gaining and losing tax the body. There's a limit to all elasticity. Eventually the stretched-out skin loses its "snap back" and becomes flab. Never take your weight for granted. Be constantly watchful to keep it just right.

Remember always that, with time, the tendency is for pounds to creep *on,* rarely off. One becomes more self-indulgent. The girl who played tennis, danced all night, walked miles with her adoring beau changes gradually into the woman who plays bridge, sits watching TV, and never walks when she can ride. If you must cut down on your activities, make a corresponding cut in calories—but do be sure to include some physical exercise as part of your life plan.

The woman of ideal weight should—after her thirtieth

birthday—replace some of the carbohydrates in her diet with protein. Small measures are often all that is needed to avoid the encroachment of pounds: for example, giving up sugar in coffee, having a salad for lunch instead of a sandwich, nibbling a raw carrot in mid-afternoon instead of cookies, replacing sweet desserts with fresh fruit. And she should weigh herself every morning, at the same hour, nude or in the same degree of undress. Weight exactly at normal? Hold to the usual design for living. The slightest bit over? Even if it's half a pound, take the immediate measure of reducing calories that day. Under normal? Don't go wild, but allow yourself a little extra treat for good behavior!

THE ZIG-ZAG DIET

Now—confession time! Reluctant as I am to admit it, I, too, sometimes gain a few extra pounds. It mostly happens when I am on an extended business trip and find myself at many elaborate luncheons and cocktail and dinner parties. The menus are often filled with regional dishes prepared especially for my enjoyment. Or it may happen right in New York, when day after day business lunches are followed by social evenings with calories whirling as fast as the pace! When the needle on the scale moves up, I go on my favorite seven-day Zig-Zag Diet. With Zig-Zag, I eat three regular meals (with normal restraint) on Zig days and very sparingly on Zag (or alternating) days. The final day I take liquids only.

This is an excellent diet for the woman of basically normal weight who needs to shed a few "new" pounds before they become entrenched. Since each day of rigid dieting is sandwiched between days of relatively normal eating, there is minimum demand on willpower. And since the diet is high in protein, it provides sufficient energy for a

MALA RUBINSTEIN'S SEVEN-DAY ZIG-ZAG DIET

	ZIG		ZAG
	MONDAY		**TUESDAY**
Breakfast	Grapefruit juice 1 poached egg 1 slice toast (no butter) Black coffee	**Breakfast**	Half grapefruit Black coffee
		11:00 A.M.	Tomato juice with lemon or hot bouillon 1 piece Melba toast
Lunch	Broiled filet of sole Grilled tomato Green salad	**Lunch**	Cottage cheese (skim-milk type) mixed with 1 stalk celery
Dinner	Roast beef (trim fat) Broccoli Small baked potato Strawberries with yogurt		diced, garnished with radish slices, in lettuce cup
		Dinner	Small lean steak, broiled Grilled tomato Green beans Cucumber salad
	WEDNESDAY		**THURSDAY**
Breakfast	Orange juice Whole-grain cereal with skim milk Black coffee	**Breakfast**	Half grapefruit Black coffee
		11:00 A.M.	Tomato juice or bouillon
Lunch	Chef's salad 1 slice pumpernickel bread 1 pat of butter Jello	**Lunch**	Tuna fish (water- packed *only*) chopped with 1 stalk of celery in lettuce cup. Flavor with lemon
Dinner	Clear soup Roast chicken Asparagus (no dressing—flavor with lemon) Rice 1 piece fresh fruit	**Dinner**	Calves liver Spinach—sea- soned with nutmeg and lemon Carrots

ZIG		ZAG	
	FRIDAY		SATURDAY
Breakfast	Stewed prunes (unsweetened) 1 boiled egg	**Breakfast**	Half grapefruit Black coffee
	1 slice buttered toast	**11:00 A.M.**	Tomato juice or bouillon
	Black coffee	**Lunch**	Half cantaloupe, cavity filled with
Lunch	Hot vegetable plate —1 cup each peas, mushrooms,		cottage cheese
	zucchini, carrots 1 slice protein	**Dinner**	Broiled halibut brussels sprouts
	bread, butter		with lemon Stewed tomato
Dinner	Small green salad 2 broiled lamb chops (small, lean) Small boiled potato Sherbet		

SUNDAY

Liquids only.

On arising —a large glass of hot water with the juice of half a lemon
Black coffee

Noon —Vegetable juice—8 oz., or hot bouillon—1 cup

5 P.M. —Tomato juice—8 oz., or grapefruit juice—8 oz.

On retiring —glass of skim milk or buttermilk

NOTE: Drink as much water as you like—but positively no alcoholic beverages.

In everyone's life there are times when three or four consecutive days of heavy eating are unavoidable. It may happen around the holidays, on vacation, or when several big social functions follow without a break. When this occurs, regardless of what the scale may read, I spend the first available day on a liquid diet. It's a good refresher for the entire system.

normal working routine. I can lose a minimum of three pounds in one week on Zig-Zag—and, best of all, at the end of the week I feel brighter and better than I did when I started.

With the exception of black coffee with breakfast, beverages are not taken with meals on Zig-Zag. Clear tea with lemon only, or black coffee, may be taken mid-afternoon. A glass of warm skim milk before retiring for the night should be taken on both Zig and Zag days. On Zig or Zag—no second helping on anything, no appetizers before dinner, no bread with dinner! On Zig days, one drink before dinner or one glass of wine with dinner is permitted. *No* liquor on Zag days!

THE WORKING WOMAN'S LUNCH

Eating lunch away from home five days a week has thrown many a diet into a tailspin (and many a body into excess poundage). Fast foods and sandwiches, the easiest choices, generally have far more calories and less good-food value than you want. A restaurant lunch may be too heavy for every day. Health bars are a kind of oasis but are not always in sight. What's a working woman to do? *Brown bag it!*

If your company provides a lounge for eating and a refrigerator for convenience, you're all set. If not, you've still got choices. You can close your office door, put a pretty place mat on your desk, switch to a different mind pattern, and enjoy lunch there. Better yet, you can take your brown bag to the nearby park bench and enjoy lunch al fresco. "Lunch out" can be pleasant, nutritious, and low in calories. Here are some ways to do it:

MAKE IT ENJOYABLE. Share your lunch hour with a friend. You might also share ideas about easy-to-carry foods that keep several hours without refrigeration.

MAKE IT ATTRACTIVE. Treat yourself to a good-looking carrier—basket, lunchbox, whatever. Stock up with colorful paper napkins, plastic forks and knives, plastic or glass containers, a thermos if you want hot consommé or a hot beverage on occasion. If you can find a small cooler, great!

MAKE IT NUTRITIOUS. If you're taking a sandwich, use whole wheat or pumpernickel bread. Make it up the night before and leave it in the freezing compartment of your refrigerator until you head for work the next day. By lunchtime, it will have thawed just enough for eating. Roast beef is a good choice. In the morning, add tomato slices (they don't freeze well) and enjoy at noon.

Don't get in a sandwich rut. Chop up leftover cooked vegetables, add a pinch of dill, a teaspoon of low-fat vegetable oil, and mix well. Store in a plastic container or glass jar to enjoy for lunch with crackers and cheese.

You can put all sorts of things in plastic containers or jars, and eat right out of the container you mix it in. Tear up salad greens. Add sliced radishes, sliced fresh mushrooms, sliced raw zucchini (any or all) and crumble roquefort cheese into the mixture. A squeeze of lemon is all the dressing you need. Another mix-and-eat concoction is shredded raw carrot and a teaspoon of raisins, mixed with your own sour cream dressing (one tablespoon of sour cream thinned with one tablespoon of skim milk).

Make your lunch a small (single serving) can of tuna fish or salmon, with celery and carrot sticks and melba toast; follow with dates and raisins. Or try slices of boned chicken, along with small cherry tomatoes and an apple for dessert.

A hard-boiled egg, melba toast, and a large orange make another good choice.

Skim milk is your best luncheon beverage. (It provides both calcium and refreshment for only 85 calories.) If you can't refrigerate or buy it nearby at lunchtime, take a small can of vegetable juice, tomato juice, or apple juice with you.

There's an important side benefit to taking your own lunch. As well as saving money, you save all the time you would otherwise spend waiting on a cafeteria line or for service in a restaurant. Use that time for a brisk walk or to exercise for half an hour if there's a health club or other facility nearby. Your lunch break can be a "lucky break" for your body—and create the livelier way you feel all afternoon!

ADDING CURVES

Slender is lovely. Scrawny is not. The woman who is too thin, too angular for body beauty is very much in the minority and, unfortunately, receives little sympathy. Overweight friends, convinced they have far more complex problems feel that all "Slim" has to do is eat an extra piece of chocolate cake and her worries are over. It's not as simple as that.

The underweight woman is not consuming enough calories to balance her energy output—or she is burning up calories too fast in nervous energy. If her appetite is poor, she faces as much difficulty in forcing herself to eat as her heavier friend does in resisting. If she's a "picky" eater, or grabs a bite on the run, or skips meals from time to time, her body mechanism can be upset to the point where she sleeps badly, feels tense, has a "knot" in her stomach, is less inclined to eat—and so it goes in a truly vicious cycle.

Attacking the problem at the source is the best approach. A little introspection is needed. You're racing your motor, but why? Some factors that lead to overweight in one woman—stress, discontent, emotional upset—may lead to underweight in another. Take time for meditation. Is the frantic rush necessary or is it your way of outpacing a problem? Make up your mind to find tranquillity in what may appear to be a sea of turmoil. Serenity is not necessarily one of life's built-in qualities. If you don't come by it naturally, seek and cultivate it. One overly thin woman I know was advised to set aside fifteen minutes before dinner to sit quietly reading poetry. She calls it her metered aperitif, and it has improved her appetite as it has calmed her nerves. Another thin girl gets similar results by grabbing the evening paper and devouring the gossip column. She's also able to entertain her friends by recounting the juiciest items of the day.

To add attractive curves to your figure, follow these basic rules:

1. Eat three ample meals each day.

2. Allow sufficient time for each meal. Get up earlier, if necessary, to enjoy a hearty breakfast. If you're a career woman, don't try to crowd shopping and errands into your lunch hour. Make a leisurely ritual out of all your meals.

3. Eat slowly, chew thoroughly.

4. Have a nourishing mid-morning and mid-afternoon snack—milk and crackers, perhaps—at least two hours before your regular meal. Before bed, drink a glass of warm milk with Ovaltine, chocolate mix, or a spoonful of honey added.

5. Cut down on stimulants. Drink milk instead of coffee or tea, when you can. Switch to decaffeinated coffee.

6. If you smoke, try to break the habit. If you can't stop completely, cut down. Never smoke immediately before a meal or between courses.

7. Keep regular sleeping hours. Eight of them every night.

8. Exercise daily to release tension, to build and shape your body.

9. Take long, leisurely walks in the fresh air to boost your appetite.

10. Have some fun. Go dancing, join a club, make a new friend, take up a new hobby. However you find it, sheer enjoyment is the greatest appetizer in the world.

11. Cultivate an interest in food. Don't depend on ready-made, heat-and-eat fare. There is fun and creativity in cooking. Find some new recipes with a gourmet twist. Plan a new decorative table setting. Delicious food, served with versatility, will wake up your taste buds!

12. Add calories to your diet.

Now about those added calories—being underweight doesn't give carte blanche as far as food is concerned. Gorging on chocolates, soft drinks, pizza, or french fries is bad for your digestion, your complexion, your well-being—regardless of your weight. Besides, the wrong food can spoil your appetite for the nutritious kind you need—the wholesome fare that produces energy, vitality, clear skin, and solid, curvaceous flesh!

Plan your diet around protein (meat, fish, chicken), leafy greens, fruits, dairy foods (eggs, cheese, whole milk) with enough carbohydrates to add firm pounds. You have an advantage over your well-padded friends in being free to enjoy some of the vitamin- and mineral-packed delights which, because of their high caloric content, are forbidden to heavyweights: avocado, sweet potato, corn, mashed potatoes, bananas, dates, raisins, lentils, nuts. Can't you hear the sighs of envy?

Before closing this chapter on food, let's speak a few words in its praise. Food does more than sustain life and give health. Over the millenniums of civilization, eating has become a social ritual. A celebration calls for a feast. Hospitality dictates that every guest be tempted with delicious fare. Business deals are consummated over lunch. People who live alone sometimes consider their main meal a highlight of the day. Romance flourishes over candlelit suppers for two. Families are never more united than at the dinner table. No wonder the kitchen is called the heart of the home! Food often satisfies a deep emotional need. To many people, it represents security, warmth, love. Seeing, smelling, or just hearing about certain foods can evoke memories of home and the carefree days of childhood.

As a guide, a weight-gaining menu for one week follows. . .

WEIGHT-GAINING MENU

	MONDAY		TUESDAY
Breakfast	Orange juice Hot cereal with milk Toast with butter Beverage	Breakfast	Orange juice Poached egg with bacon Toast with butter Beverage
Lunch	2-egg omelette Mixed green salad Roll and butter Fresh fruit cup	Lunch	Baked macaroni with cheese and small meatballs Broccoli Fresh fruit cup
Dinner	Cream of mushroom soup Roast beef Baked potato Peas Blueberry pie	Dinner	Hearts of lettuce Fillet of sole *bonne femme* with mushrooms Carrots Rice Roll and butter Sherbet with crushed pineapple
	WEDNESDAY		THURSDAY
Breakfast	Stewed prunes Cereal with sliced banana, milk Toast with butter Beverage	Breakfast	Prune juice Stewed tomato on toast Beverage
Lunch	Vegetable plate Roll and butter Gelatin with fruit	Lunch	Vegetable soup Grilled cheese sandwich Sherbet
Dinner	Grapefruit and avocado slices Calves liver with bacon Asparagus Mashed potatoes Rice pudding	Dinner	Shrimp cocktail Baked ham Sweet potato Spinach Hot biscuit Pear Hélène

	FRIDAY		SATURDAY
Breakfast	Orange juice French toast Beverage	Breakfast	Half grapefruit Scrambled eggs with chopped ham Toast with butter Jam or marmalade Beverage
Lunch	Avocado filled with cottage cheese or chicken salad Hard roll with butter Stewed rhubarb	Lunch	Raw vegetable salad Bread and butter Ice cream
Dinner	Lettuce and tomato salad Veal chop String beans Buttered noodles Chocolate pudding	Dinner	Consommé Roast chicken Oven-browned potato Cauliflower and peas Baked apple with cream

Snacks daily, at 10:30 A.M. and 4:00 P.M., may include milk and graham crackers, fresh fruit, fresh dates, raisins, raw vegetables. Before bed, drink a glass of warm milk with a spoonful of honey or chocolate syrup.

FOOD FOR THOUGHT—AND BEAUTY

When I was growing up in Kraków, our kitchen was redolent with the aroma of homemade bread, of delicious Polish specialties like zrazy and stuffed goose, of rich-filled naleśniki and pastries that seemed to melt in the mouth. And, looking back, it seems I was always able to clean my plate with gusto, yet was always thin as a rail. During my first year in Paris, I often sought out little restaurants that served the hearty Polish food for which I had developed a taste and craving. It was food with the flavor of home, and I was drawn by nostalgia as much as appetite.

Part of the intensive training planned for me at that time, in relation to beauty, included study of nutrition. From these lessons, plus my own observation, I knew that my childhood diet was no longer suitable for my life, activities—and looks. Of course, the superb French cuisine to which I was newly exposed—the delectable sauces, the seven- and eight-course dinners, the magnificent desserts—also offered great temptation. I knew that I must adopt a new approach to food. Gradually, I learned to make the rich foods I loved rare treats instead of regular fare. I learned to enjoy the nourishing, energy-giving, less calorie-laden dishes. And I learned to take smaller portions.

From now on, be more aware of what you eat—not merely the taste, but what the food and drink does *to* and *for* your body. Think in terms of vitamins, minerals, calories. Change your food shopping habits if necessary. Become a label-reader. Prepared foods often contain more salt, sugar, chemical preservatives than you want to include in your diet. Learn which to avoid, what you can substitute, how to eat creatively rather than destructively.

When I visited the famous Bircher-Benner Institute in Switzerland, under the guidance of the great nutritionist Dr. Bircher-Benner, I became aware not only of the principles but of the *joy* of eating for health and long-lasting youthfulness. I've been an advocate of Food for Beauty ever since.

Changing one's eating habits is difficult, but when the change is for the better the rewards are great. When you choose Food for Beauty gladly and truly consider it *beautiful* food, you'll have reached the right mental attitude—and it will all be reflected in a more vital, more attractive YOU.

BEAUTY IN MOTION

Exercise is for *everybody*. It's not a question of choice; it's essential for your health and beauty. To me it's one of the truly enjoyable essentials of life. It can be for everyone. It's a matter of mental attitude—of finding the kinds of exercise that give you the most fun—and of experiencing the rewards (which are pleasure-inducing indeed).

There's joy in motion. Watch a gull soar across the sky, a horse canter in a meadow, children at play. You can recapture the same exhilarating sensation with exercise and at the same time improve your appearance and well-being. Are you aware of all the things accomplished by controlled body motion? Teamed with sensible diet, it assures a well-proportioned, trim, firm figure. It gives strength and grace. It dispels nervous tension. It aids the circulation, the digestion, the functioning of the fantastic internal mechanism. A vivacious French star once told me that she attributed her tremendous *joie de vivre* (on which I had just complimented her) to good blood circulation. She had a point! I've personally witnessed the transformation of many personalities from flat ale to bubbling champagne when exercise became a health-making habit. And here's another good reason for it—doctors tell us that regular exercise, combined with nutritious food, is a prime factor in keeping the body young. Age, like moss, gathers on the motionless stone!

To be effective, however, exercise must be part of your daily design. Yes, *daily*. A burst of activity, followed by a long coast, doesn't work. The benefits of exercise can't be stored away for use when needed. You'll see and feel results only when exercise is a well-regulated habit. Once you have made it so, you'll find it as indispensable as your morning coffee—but more invigorating and far better for you.

Enjoy sports as often as you can. Take up a new one now and then, adapted to the vigor your age and condition permit. Swimming, tennis, skating, golf, bicycling are all exhilarating, delightful and good physical exercise. Rediscover your feet. Put them in comfortable, low-heeled shoes and take a long, brisk walk daily. Dance around your room to the strains of your favorite music. And by all means make calisthenics part of your daily schedule; it's the best way of assuring controlled movement of various parts of your body, of toning and reshaping as needed.

Find delight in motion. It's one of the great sensory

pleasures, and anyone who misses out on it is cheating himself not only of the physical rewards but also of the sheer fun it brings. Even fun has ground rules, however, and here are a few to keep in mind if you want to wring the utmost in enjoyment and effectiveness from your exercise:

. . .Before you start vigorous exercising or take up an active new sport, get your doctor's okay. This is especially important if you've been leading a sedentary life.
. . .Decide where and when you will exercise. Set aside a definite time.
. . .Get an exercise mat (a large beach towel or blanket will serve) and keep it accessible. You'll need it for the on-the-floor routines.
. . .Wear suitable exercise clothes. Buy yourself the prettiest leotards you can find (you'll enjoy the daily session that much more) or wear a bathing suit, bikini, or other outfit that allows free motion. Barefoot is best—or just socks.
. . .Move to music—your favorite kind, whatever it may be.
. . .Work into your schedule gradually. If you've been inactive, five minutes of exercise will be enough the first two or three days, then ten minutes a day for the balance of the week. Work up to twenty or thirty minutes a day if you are trying to firm flabby areas or improve your measurements. Once the tape says "great!" fifteen minutes daily, coupled with walks and sports, is adequate.
. . .Exercise *daily* for the rest of your life. Never ever let your body become the victim of your indolence!

Doing the same set of exercises every day of the week, every week of the year, is as boring as having turkey for dinner every night or wearing the same dress every day. And it's not necessary. The world is full of exercises—isometric, classic, Yoga, Chinese, ad infinitum. Like recipes, they can be clipped from magazines and kept on tile, some for future reference. There are basic patterns and there are many variations on those patterns, which bring into play areas of the body that may have been relatively neglected. Each session should include exercises for *all* parts of your body. Working for an hour on leg exercises isn't going to firm flabby upper arms or ward off a double chin. Exercising every body area not only keeps you toned all over, but helps circulation and flexibility. I'm going to give you a number of exercises—grouped according to their type. You may want to try them first in context, but then do juggle them around, mix them up, plan a whole new "menu" now and then, for your greater enjoyment and for greater rewards.

WARM-UP "ISOLATIONS"

This is a routine to "warm-up" the body, each part in isolation, before proceeding to exercises for specific purpose. Repeat each one four to six times. In standing position:

Head	Slowly nod back and forth. Nod sideways, leaning the ear toward the shoulder on one side, then the other side.
Neck	Roll the head slowly in a circle from right to left, left to right.
Shoulders	Raise both shoulders as high as you can. Hold for six-count. Drop as low as possible. Rotate shoulders forward, then backward.
Arms and Chest	With elbows bent and held out at right angles to body, touch the fingertips of one hand to the other at chest level. Be sure chest is held high. Now fling arms

out as wide as possible, throwing head
back at the same time. Return to position.

Hands and Wrists Extend arms straight out in front, palms
down. Turn hands upward from the
wrist, holding them at right angles to
the arm. Then curl them under, trying
to touch inside of wrist with fingertips.
Relax hands and wiggle all fingers.

Diaphragm   Hands on hips, thrust rib cage forward,
now push the rib cage to the right, to the
back, to the left. Try not to move any
other part of the body.

Waist   Hands on hips, roll the body around in a
circle from the waist, first in one direc-
tion, then the other.

Hips   Bend one knee; bring it as close as you
can to the chest. Repeat with the other
knee. Motion should come *from the hip;*
let the hip lift the knee and leg.

Thighs   Feet wide apart, hands on hips, push the
right hip out as far as possible and shift
weight to the right side, pressing against the side with a bouncing motion.
Feel the pressure on the inner thigh.
Switch to left side and repeat.

Ankles   Balance on one foot, raise the other
slightly and circle the ankle from right
to left, left to right. Change to other foot
and repeat.

BEAUTY DOZEN

Twelve basic exercises, to do daily, that will keep the entire body well-toned and graceful. Run through the entire routine, then repeat those that apply to areas of special need.

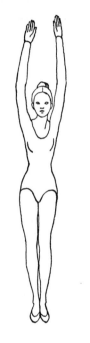

1. For Arms and Overall Toning

Stand with feet together, arms up. Stretch one arm after the other toward the ceiling, reaching as high as you can. Ten times.

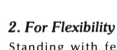

2. For Flexibility

Standing with feet about 12" apart, stretch backward and forward from the waist, arms following the body. Ten times.

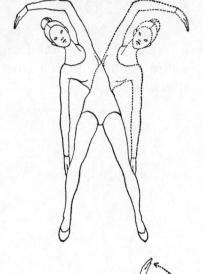

3. To Whittle Your Waist

Stretch as far as you can to the right side, curving your left arm over your head—reach and stretch hard with the arm. Reverse to other side. Six to eight times each side.

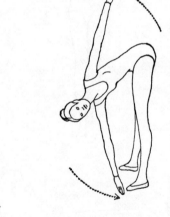

4. For Waist, Back, Shoulders, Arms

Feet apart, stretch from the waist and touch right toe with left hand, swinging your other arm back at the same time. Now swing the right hand down to touch the left toe, as the left arm swings back. Eight to twelve times each side.

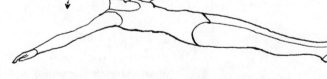

5. For Neck Muscles and "Dowager's Hump"

Lie on floor, arms stretched out at shoulder level, palms up. Lift head and shoulders and pull chin toward chest, keeping hands on floor. Return head very slowly. Six to eight times.

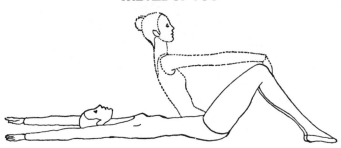

6. To Help Firm Abdomen

Flat on back, knees bent, feet on floor, arms overhead—slowly raise head and upper body. Touch knees with hands and roll back. Six to eight times.

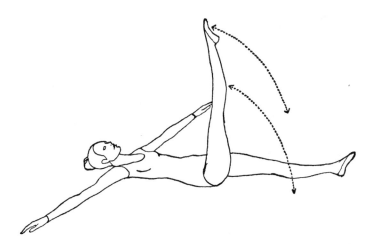

7. For Toning Thighs

Flat on back, arms stretched at shoulder level. Pick up left leg until it is at right angles to the body. With knee straight, cross leg to the right side, touching the floor, then bring it back. Repeat with same leg six to eight times, then reverse to the other leg.

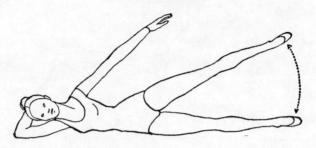

8. To Help Firm Inner Thigh

Lie on right side, head resting on arm. Lift left leg, knee straight, as high as possible. Kick up and down eight to twelve times. Reverse to left side, right leg.

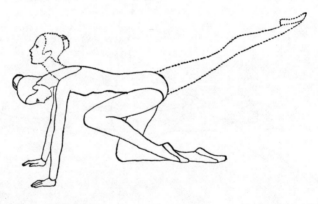

9. For Back, Hips, Throat

Start on hands and knees, with back straight. Drop head and bring the right knee slowly forward, trying to touch your nose. Feel the stretch in your spine. Bring the leg back, stretching it straight out behind. Reverse to other leg. Four to six times with each leg.

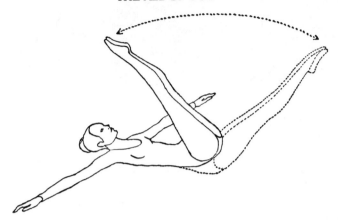

10. For Back and Flexibility

Lie on floor, arms stretched out at shoulder level. Lift both legs, toes pointing toward ceiling. Sway legs back toward your head, lifting lower back off the floor. Sway back and forth ten times.

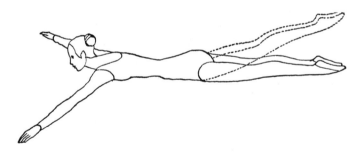

11. For Derriere, Stomach, Legs

Lie stomach-down on floor. Lift both legs, keeping them together with knees straight, as high as you can. Hold for count of five, then drop them slowly back. Four to six times.

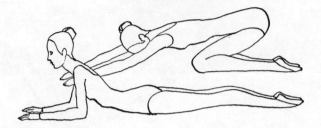

12. For Hips, Back

Stretch out on floor, hands supporting body under shoulders; elbows bent, legs together. Straightening arms, push torso back as far as possible. Thrust torso forward again, as you straighten knees. Six to eight times.

BEAUTY STRETCH EXERCISES

Watch a cat awaken. Ah-h-h, that long, luxurious, sensuous stretch—from the tip of its pink nose to the last hair of its tail. It's a motion that looks as though it must feel delightful—and it does. Try it and see. Stretching is one of the most enjoyable motions of all and, while you savor the pleasure in each inch of you, that long pull is toning the muscles, easing any tightness or nervous tension, making your body more supple and lithe. The most valuable stretches are done very slowly, as each part of your body reaches, reaches, reaches for something just a little beyond your touch.

Stretching exercises are my favorites. They can be done almost anywhere, almost anytime. Seated in a plane, train or car, you can give your torso a good pull upward from base of spine to neck—then give your head an upward stretch; you can raise your legs, one after the other, and give each a slow stretch; you can hold arms at your sides and reach downward, then raise and stretch to the ceiling. At the office, you can do the same thing—then spread out your arms as if you're trying to touch the wall on either side as you feel a wonderful resilience through your shoulders right down to your fingertips.

When I exercise at home, I use an elasticized rope which I believe helps me to get the greatest benefit from every motion. As a matter of fact, I keep it under my pillow and immediately upon arising I have a few "good morning" stretches to get the day off to a happy start. Here are a few of my favorite Beauty Stretch exercises:

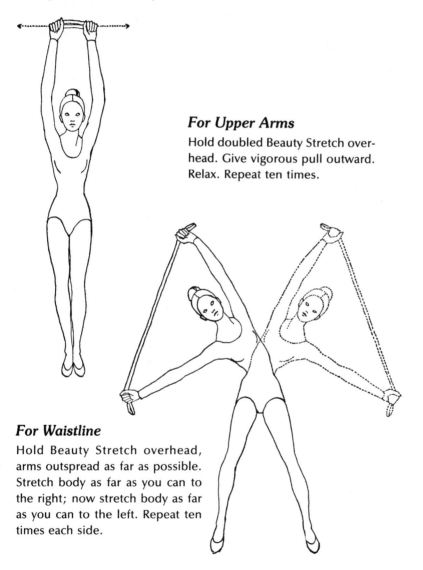

For Upper Arms

Hold doubled Beauty Stretch overhead. Give vigorous pull outward. Relax. Repeat ten times.

For Waistline

Hold Beauty Stretch overhead, arms outspread as far as possible. Stretch body as far as you can to the right; now stretch body as far as you can to the left. Repeat ten times each side.

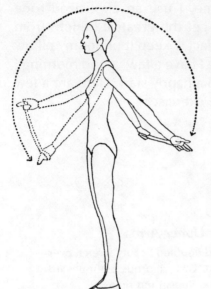

For Upper Arms, Shoulders, "Dowager's Hump"

Hold Beauty Stretch in hands, arms dropped in back and spread as far apart as possible. Raise arms up, over head, forward and down. Reverse, bringing arms up, over head and back. Hands must be as far apart as possible throughout. Repeat ten times.

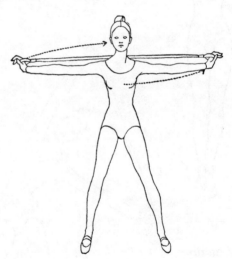

For Waistline

Stand erect, feet apart, Beauty Stretch held behind, resting on shoulder blades, arms straight. Swing upper torso, from the waist, as far as you can to the right; swing as far left as you can. Keep swinging ten times in each direction.

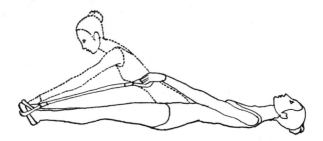

For Stomach and Back

Sit on floor. Loop Beauty Stretch over each instep, holding center in both hands. Roll back very slowly, until head touches floor. Pull on Beauty Stretch to roll up and forward, touching hands to toes. Repeat six times.

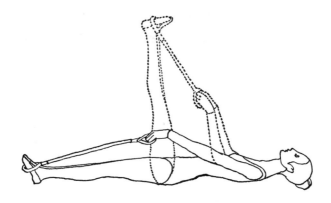

For The Upper Legs and Calves

Same position as for previous exercise. Keep torso on floor and, holding center of Beauty Stretch, bring legs straight up and slowly lower them without bending knees. Repeat four to six times.

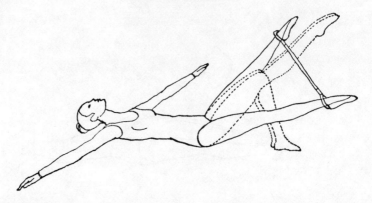

For The Thighs

Loop Beauty Stretch over insteps. Lie on floor, arms outstretched at shoulder level, knees bent, feet on floor. Straighten legs and stretch them to ceiling. Now, open legs wide to full extent of Beauty Stretch. Close legs, bend knees and bring feet to floor. Repeat four to six times.

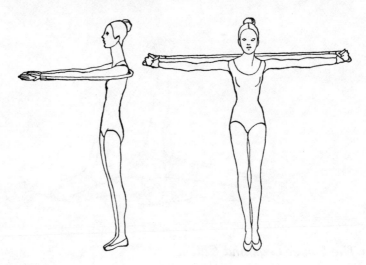

For The Chest, Throatline, and Upper Arms

Slip hands into loops of Beauty Stretch. Slip it back over your shoulders, letting it rest on shoulder blades. Now extend arms, keeping elbows straight, to shoulder level and bring palms together. Separate hands slowly until arms are at wingspread position, thrusting chin out. Bring palms together and repeat six times.

THE LAZY WOMAN'S EXERCISES—
THE EARLY MORNING TEN

There goes the alarm—and she just can't get up. That five minutes more in bed means five minutes less time to get dressed and out of the house—and, too often, it means no time for exercise. If this happens to *you* make "The Lazy Woman's Exercises" part of your morning routine. They are designed to be done before you get out of bed with a minimum of space, preparation, and time. If you practice these "waker uppers" *every* morning, they'll help you to keep trim and give your day a better start, too!

1. First, toss your pillow aside and take a good all-over stretch. Curl your right arm over your head and stretch the entire right side right down to your toes. Curl your left arm over your head and stretch that side. Throw arms out at shoulder level and stretch again.
2. Lying flat, arms at sides, raise your head *only* up and down a few times.
3. Throw the covers back and raise the upper part of your body, bending forward from the waist to touch your toes. Reach beyond them if you can. Return to flat position by "unfolding" vertebra by vertebra until your head touches the bed. Repeat six to eight times.
4. Lie flat. Raise your left leg until it is at right angles to the body and return it to place. Repeat eight times with left leg; eight times with right leg.
5. Turn on your right side and lift the left leg straight up and down eight times. Turn on left side and lift the right leg up and down eight times.
6. Lie on your back with knees bent, feet flat. Keeping your back on the bed, lift your hips and pelvis as high as you can, hold for a moment, return. Repeat six times.
7. Lie with head and upper part of your shoulders hanging over the bottom of the bed (if there is no footboard;

otherwise lie across the bed with head and shoulders over the side). Throw your arms back so that they are hanging down, out of the bed and over your head; now raise your arms, head, and upper part of your body, touching your hands in front of you. Return to first position. With this exercise breathe in deeply as you come up, breathe out as you go down. Repeat six times.

8. Sit upright in bed, legs straight but held as far apart as possible. Swing from the waist to touch the left toe with your right hand, swinging left arm behind you at the same time. Keep arms straight! Now swing to touch the right toe with your left hand. Keep swinging rhythmically, like a windmill, eight to twelve times.

9. In the same position—upright with legs straight but far apart—grasp your left ankle with your left hand, left knee with your right hand. Pull your upper body down toward your leg, trying to touch it with your left ear. Give six to eight pulling "bounces." Repeat on the right side.

10. Now even the laziest girl is ready to get out of bed. Sit on the side, back straight, and fold your hands on your chest, elbows out and up, head down. Now throw the arms out as far as you can and raise your head at the same time. Return arms and head to starting position. Repeat eight times please.

Simple weren't they? And in just five minutes you've exercised for waist, back, thighs, hips, arms, chest, throat, and chin, as well as over-all body toning. Even an active woman might want to add this "Early Morning Ten" to her daily routine!

COPING-WITH-THE-WORLD EXERCISES
(For sheer relaxation)

> The world is too much with us; late and soon,
> Getting and spending, we lay waste our powers. . . .

Too true, Mr. Wordsworth, too true. When the world seems to be pressing in, when the day has come to a calamitous end, when you feel desperately driven—be driven, not to the old demon, but to the kind of exercise that encourages relaxation. Tension, which can knot up the entire body, is concentrated along the spine where all the tender nerve endings are housed. A great many people tell me they "get it in the neck," both figuratively and literally! There are some wonderful ways to relieve this build-up of tension, especially helpful at the end of a busy day to revitalize, refresh, and restore your bounce before an evening of pleasurable pursuits.

1. THE TRANQUILIZER
If you are extremely tense but have a big evening ahead, do this one first and follow with the others. If you want to release tension only so that you may get to bed and have a good night's sleep, do this one last.

Lie on a hard surface (preferably the floor). No pillow—but roll a small towel and place it under your neck. Raise your feet on pillows. Close your eyes and try to clear your mind of all thought. Breathe rhythmically—and let it be *abdominal breathing.* Push out the abdominal wall as you breathe in, draw in the abdomen as you exhale. Breathe slowly; become absorbed in the rhythm. Now think consciously of your tense muscles and relax them one by one, starting at your toes and working slowly up to the top of your head. Give each a gentle command, "Toes—relax," "Ankles—relax," "Calves—relax," and up and up. Keep your eyes closed all the time and little by little you will feel tension slipping away.

2. THE UNKNOTTER

When you're "in knots," try this one. Lie on the floor, completely flat, arms at sides. Slowly raise your legs, keeping both together, lifting the lower spine off the floor and bringing your legs parallel with your body. Think of being a U on its side. Support your lower back with your hands, if necessary. Stay in this position for a minute or two, then slowly return to flat.

3. THE REVIVER

Again flat on your back. Raise your legs *up* this time, holding them together, until you are resting your weight almost completely on your shoulders and the rest of your body is in a vertical line. Hold it there as long as you can. Support your body with your hands and arms until you are so controlled that you can perform this shoulder stand "no hands." This is an especially good exercise if you've been on your feet all day, and if you want to renew your energy for hours ahead.

4. THE RAG DOLL

Stand with feet twelve inches apart. Let your body drop forward from the waist, head and arms limp. Now, from the lower spine, bounce a little so that your limp body flops up and down—directly in front, then flopping to the side so that your body is over the right foot, slowly flopping over to the left foot and return. "Flop" at least twelve times, then *slowly* raise your body, starting at the base of the spine and working up vertebra by vertebra until you are completely upright. Raise arms upward and "climb" by raising one hand after the other, each reaching as high as possible. Repeat.

5. FOR HEAD AND SHOULDER TENSION (sit in a chair to do these)

a) Fixing your eyes on an object straight ahead of you, bend your head as far as possible toward your right shoulder. Hold it for a moment, then straighten it. Repeat on the left side. Do this two or three times on each side.

b) Lift your forehead as high as your eyebrows will go. Feel your scalp "lifting." Hold for count of three. Relax. Repeat several times.

c) Let your head fall forward, then roll it slowly in an arc from left shoulder to right shoulder and back. Then rotate it slowly in a complete circle. Reverse.

d) Sitting erect, lean forward from your hips. Place hands on your shoulders, elbows straight out. Now bring the elbows up and back, trying to touch elbow to elbow behind your head. Bring elbows down to sides. Be sure to keep hands on your shoulders throughout.

e) Lift one shoulder as high as possible. Hold for count of three. Drop. Now do the same thing with the other shoulder. Repeat several times on each side.

6. THE UNINHIBITED DANCE
Put on some lively music—jazz, rock, bouzouki, flamenco—and give it all you've got! Be a go-go, a twister, a belly dancer, a Spanish gypsy. Move as the spirit moves you. Get your arms, your shoulders, your whole body, into the act as well as your legs. If the tempo demands it, give a frustration-crushing stamp now and then. If the man downstairs complains, invite him to join you in a paso doble. Dancing is one of the best relaxants, especially when it's "free form."

MAKE EVERY MOTION COUNT
Do you know that you can get a beauty "bonus" by incorporating exercise into many routine activities? The day is made up of a thousand details—and motions without number. If you make bad posture and careless movement a habit, at the end of each day you will be just a little closer to a sagging figure. If, however, you maintain perfect posture and use your body properly, you'll feel less tired, be more controlled in your posture, and will have made many moves

toward a more shapely figure. Use your imagination to find the many ways you can exercise as you move through the day. Here are a few to start with:

Bathe beautifully with stretching motions that help your waistline. . .

Sit tall to wash your back; reach far down your back with one arm, then with the other. Keep legs outstretched and reach from the waist to wash ankles and toes. Between latherings, place the soap just out of reach so that you must stretch for it.

Dance as you dry your shoulders and arms. . .

Hum a Latin American tune and hold the towel tight as you slide it back and forth.

Stretch with right arm, then with left as you move the towel from shoulder, down back. Give a few hip wiggles, too.

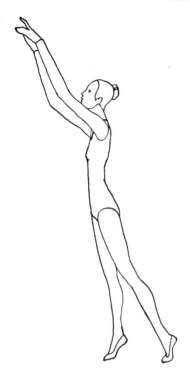

Reach the highest shelf and help tone body and arms. . .
As you reach up, tuck your pelvis under, place one leg behind the other, go up on your toes and give a good, all-over *s-t-r-e-t-c-h.*

Weed the garden or go to the lowest file . . . you'll grow posture perfect, firm up thighs. . .
Keep your back arrow-straight and with one foot a little in front of the other, lower yourself from your hips. When you rise, don't tip forward. Let the thighs do the work to raise you straight up, with full weight on the balls of your feet.

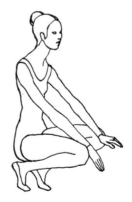

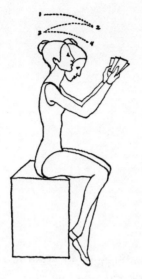

Win at bridge, work off a dowager's hump, work on a slim midriff. . .

Pull up from your diaphragm and bring cards level with your eyes. This is the correct sitting position. Hold it as long as you can. While cards are being dealt, relieve tension (and dowager's hump) by tossing head back as far as possible, then dropping chin to chest.

Take a break from desk work or TV viewing. . .

Makes your back supple, slims your arms, firms your chin line. . . Stretch your fingers to the ceiling, toes to the floor, back straight— your whole body making a V. Now throw your head back and stretch your arms out at shoulder level, reaching out as far as you can.

POSTURE—VITAL KEY
TO BODY BEAUTY

Posture creates an *immediate* impression—favorable or not.
Correct posture is the basis of figure beauty.
Good posture gives a better figure *instantly.*
The habit of good posture promises a lovelier,
young-looking figure for *life!*

"You sound positively evangelistic," someone told me,
after I had finished preaching good posture to a group of
college seniors. I had been programmed to talk on the
psychological effect of cosmetics. However, as I was
introduced to my audience, I was appalled to see how they
were slumped, sprawled, and twisted in their chairs. The
faces were young, fresh, bright, yet their bodies were being
misused in a manner that would produce unattractive
shapes in later years. A lovely head was jutting forward; in
time this would be a permanent pose, with a slack wedge of
flesh under the chin. The girl with rounded shoulders was
working up to a Uriah Heep stance. Those who slumped
would complain, in a few years, of chronic backache. The
many who let their bodies "fold down" in unattractive sags
would have permanent "accordion pleats" around their
middles. Before I could start my scheduled talk, I had the
girls rise while I instructed them in perfect standing
position. Then I showed them how to sit gracefully,
comfortably, beautifully. If I lectured them with fervor on
the subject of posture, it was heartfelt, and I know that
those who were inspired to practice good posture found the
instruction as valuable as the scheduled talk on psychology
which followed—and perhaps more applicable to their lives.
The way you carry your body helps to shape it. The
effect may be slow, but it is certainly steady. Look around
at any group of middle-aged people and you will see at a

glance who made a habit of good posture and who underes-
timated its importance. I love to see young girls carry
themselves proudly; they become magnificent in appearance. But most of all I enjoy the shining example of women
who, through the habit of good posture through the years,
look vital, confident, more attractive at *every* age.

Good posture makes a world of difference in one's
appearance. Try it and see. Observe yourself in your
natural stance in a full-length mirror. (Better yet, when
you catch your image in an unguarded moment, take a good
look at yourself.) This is how others see you.
Now—straighten up. Pull your stomach in, tuck your
derrière under, hold your chest high, shoulders back but
relaxed, head straight on your spine with chin parallel to
floor. Have a second look. Don't you seem pounds lighter,
years younger, more vibrantly alive? This is the posture
which you must maintain always. Remind yourself,
throughout the day, to stand, sit, and walk "tall." Your
spine is a long cord; try to imagine someone pulling it from
above your head making it as straight as possible. Pretend
your whole body is being lifted up—up—your feet barely
touching the ground. At first it may be an effort. Gradually
it will be automatic. Perfect posture is a good exercise in
itself. Each time you pull your stomach in, you are helping
to firm and flatten that middle area. Each time you
straighten your back you are helping your spine. Each time
you hold your rib cage high rather than letting it sag into
the abdominal area, you are giving all your internal organs
a break. Since good posture actually strengthens the
supportive muscles, the longer and more conscientiously
you practice it, the easier it is to maintain.

Have you seen women with lovely standing posture
who lose it when they "dump" themselves into a chair? To
sit properly, approach the chair and, with your back to
it—the back of one leg actually touching it, one foot
somewhat in front of the other—lower yourself into the

seat. Keep your head high and back straight. Your weight will be on your legs. And don't steer with your derrière; keep it tucked under. When you sit, keep the small of your back pressed against your chair, rib cage held high, stomach in, head straight on your spine. When you lean forward, do it from the waist. And keep legs *together* please! Sit with feet flat on floor or with one foot just in front of the other. If you cross your legs, cross at the ankles—not at the knees—alternating to avoid stiffness and poor circulation.

When you walk, check all posture points—and be sure your toes point straight ahead. Primary action in walking should come from the thigh. Arms should be relaxed. Let them follow the body naturally. As you stride, breathe in deeply to the count of four steps, hold your breath for the count of the next four, breathe out for the count of the following four. Notice how this breathing exercise helps you to keep good posture.

When you climb stairs, keep your head high and your back straight. Place the ball of your foot on the step and lift yourself by using your thigh muscles. Don't let your derrière jut out in back or your head poke forward in front.

Do you remember Eliza Doolittle's arrival at the ball? What a glorious moment! All conversation stopped. Heads turned. There were whispers of, "Who *is* she?" as the little cockney flower girl floated by, looking every inch a countess. However rigorously Professor Higgins had coached her in diction, could she have made this Grand Entrance without magnificent carriage? Her proud and confident bearing—the attitude of a beautiful woman— raised her status as surely as her newly refined speech did.

We can all learn from Eliza. Entrances are important; this is the moment when impressions are made, when one's self-assurance is shored up or shattered. Whether you're entering a ballroom, a friend's living room, a restaurant, or your boss's office—pause for a moment on the threshold.

Bursting into a room as if to take it by surprise attack or slithering in with a droop are both unattractive. Whenever you enter a room (*any* room) use that moment of pause to quickly review all posture points. Every entrance can't be a "grand" one, but it can be one that is good and attractive.

Good posture, faithfully practiced, becomes second nature. Holding yourself proudly and properly is the best way to achieve it. However, I do recommend that you also include some "Posture Perfect" exercises in your daily schedule. Here are a few that are designed to tune up and strengthen the supportive muscles that hold the body in a lovely line.

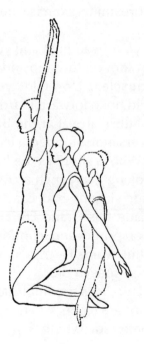

1. Seated on heels with arms at sides, back straight, lift to a kneeling position as you bring arms up from sides and reach to the ceiling. Sit down slowly without arching spine and bring arms back to sides. The hips are tucked under throughout.

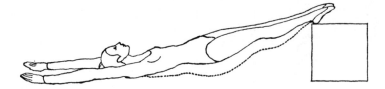

2. Lie on floor, feet resting up on bed or chair and arms stretched out on floor above head, slowly lift the hips up off the floor. Roll back to floor very slowly, bringing the small of the back down first, then the hips. Do this ten times.

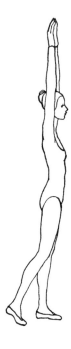

3. Hold arms straight above head; pull arms as far back as possible without arching spine. Walk around room holding this position.

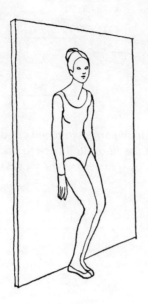

4. Stand with back, head, and shoulders against wall, arms relaxed at sides. Pull abdomen in, tilting pelvis under and bending knees just enough so that small of back touches wall. Relax. Repeat five to ten times.

5. If you tend to have an arched spine, practice walking backwards with back straight.

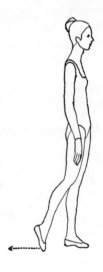

THE CARE THAT MAKES
A BODY BEAUTIFUL

On the Grecian Island of Rhodes, while I was admiring the ancient statues at the Archeological Museum, I noticed a young Englishman gazing, completely enrapt, at the fabulous Aphrodite. Since I am interested in the *effect* of beauty as well as its creation, I became engrossed in his reaction as he surveyed the statue from every angle, his eye moving along the gentle slopes and curves, a look of absolute veneration in his eyes. After a few minutes, aware I was watching him, he turned to me with a bemused expression and said, "Lovely toes, hasn't she?" As a matter of fact, she did have lovely toes. She had lovely *everything.* The young man's face was more expressive than his comment, however, and it clearly said that the beholder's eye doesn't dwell on beauty's face alone.

I don't minimize the importance of the face. After all, it is both the focal point and the most active instrument of expression. And because, unlike other parts of the anatomy, it is exposed to the elements of all seasons and subject to the ripples of every grimace, frown, and squint, it demands special attention, as does its stem—the neck. However, that doesn't relegate the rest of you to a Siberia of carelessness! Beauty is the sum of many parts—of all your parts—and each should be as perfect as you can make it. Your body is shaped and vitalized by diet and exercise; its health depends on internal factors. But to be as smooth, unblemished, and admirable as an alabaster statue, it needs loving care from the *outside,* too. Every woman who wants to feel attractive, desirable, confident, when the glance goes *below* her neck will include in her design for living these simple, but important attentions. . . .

FOR AN ALABASTER SMOOTH BODY

Your complexion covers the all of you—and your total complexion should be as smooth, even-textured, pretty as your face. Have you ever noticed—the first warm day of the season—the assorted skins that come out of hiding: mottled, dry-looking arms, flaky, unkempt legs; shoulders that deserve a "cold shoulder" in return. And then, in contrast, other bodies are as lovely as any work of art—and are often the product of their owners' artistry. Your body complexion is not as vulnerable as your face, but it *is* subject to many of the same influences—and it will respond beautifully to simple treatment.

"Why does my body skin get so dry?" many women ask me. It's our modern life style. We eat fewer fatty foods (better to be slimmer, healthier, longer-lived). We're kept comfortable by artificial heat in winter, by air conditioning in summer. We bathe daily—sometimes more frequently. We may use soap that is too harsh or drying. We expose our bodies to the sun. The result is often a dry, taut feeling which can lead to crepey, old-looking body skin. The need is for moisture and lubrication. After tub or shower, stroke a smoothing cream or lotion over your entire body. Choose one that is quickly absorbed but rich in emollients. Give special attention and a little extra lubricant to parts of the body prone to extreme dryness and roughening: the elbows, the heels, the knees.

"But my body skin feels oily—and I have pimples and blackheads on my shoulders" is another cry—often from young people. In all probability, the cause stems from the same physical condition that results in an oily face, although the manifestation is rarely as severe. Use a medicated soap to wash the body and don't skip that daily bath or shower. If there are pimples or blackheads on the shoulders or upper back, use a friction-wash on the area and touch the pimples with a healing medicated cream. However, even when the overall skin condition is relatively oily, some areas—elbows, knees, feet—are prone to dryness and should be given the lubricating care they require.

ARMS—TO HAVE AND TO HOLD

Have you ever mused on the missing arms of the Venus de Milo? How divinely proportioned they must have been; how proudly and gracefully the living model must have used them! You're starting with an advantage over Venus since you *have* yours—and whether or not they are an asset is up to you. A liability quality is flabbiness, most often noticeable in the upper arm, due to poor muscle tone, and a mottled look, due to poor circulation. Daily exercise will help both conditions. Along with your regular calisthenics, add a few stretches throughout the day to keep arms flexible, gracefully attractive in motion. Almost anytime, almost anyplace, you can stretch your arms down, out, up—reaching until you feel tension in the upper arms. Then give them a good shake. When you apply smoothing lotion to your arms, use the entire palm, with strong massaging motion. Start at the wrist and press up firmly to the shoulder.

Never lean on your elbows—at table, beach, office, anywhere. It makes them rough and horny looking. If your elbows are discolored and flaky, give them a friction-wash with the same cleansing granules recommended for deep-cleansing the face; rinse, dry, and apply a rich lubricating cream. Whenever you use lotion on your hands, rub some into your elbows, too.

I've heard many girls moan about their hairy arms; sometimes without good cause. With the rarest exceptions, all arms grow hair. It is not unattractive, or even too apparent, except when it is extremely heavy or dark. Unless it is either or both, my advice is to leave it. However, if arm hair *does* pose a problem, first consider bleaching as the solution. Lighter hair is less apparent and continued bleaching weakens the strands which is a most desirable reaction in areas where the hair itself is not wanted! As a second choice, consider removing the hair by waxing or depilation (following the same procedure as suggested for legs later in this chapter). *Never* shave your arms. The bristly regrowth will be more unattractive, more apparent than the down you started with.

Underarms, of course, must be hair free. Remove underarm hair by shaving, waxing, or depilation. Don't use a deodorant or antiperspirant for at least 24 hours after removing hair.

HANDS—LOVELY TO HOLD AND BEHOLD

As "little messengers of love," hands have inspired poets and composers. Who can forget Romeo sighing his wish to be a glove upon the hand of his Juliet? After your face, nothing is more revealing of your character—or of a fleeting mood—than your hands. Their structural form, their condition and grooming, the manner in which you use them, whisper compliments or carry cruel tales. If you want every message to be kind, follow these tips:

. . . Be sure your hands are always immaculately clean. At least once daily, scrub the nails and finger tips with a firm hand brush. Wash your hands throughout the day, as needed, with a pure mild soap. *Pat* dry (don't rub) and push the cuticle back gently with a soft towel.

. . . Smooth on hand lotion after every wetting. To ensure consistency, keep lotion wherever you wash your hands—in the bathroom, the kitchen, at the office. Keep another bottle at your bedside, so that you can smooth lotion on your hands just before slumber.

. . . Protect your hands. Use rubber gloves for dishwashing, laundry, any wet work. Use heavy fabric gloves for gardening or other hefty chores. Save your old cotton

gloves for dusting and other light tasks. Don't expose
your bare hands out-of-doors when the weather is cold
or windy. Some women, especially those who freckle,
like to protect their hands against the burning sun, too.

. . . Once weekly—more often when hands are chap-
ped—massage a rich lubricating cream into your hands
before going to bed. Start at the fingertips and "pull"
the cream down each finger, down the thumb, down the
back of the hand, as if you were drawing on a pair of
tight gloves. Work the cream around each nail, into the
cuticle. If there is a residue of creaminess, wear loose
cotton gloves to bed.

. . . Strong nails depend on inherent factors, your diet, your
physical condition. Eating gelatin, or taking the
unflavored kind daily in fruit juice, often helps weak
nails. Another aid: soak the nails (without polish) for
ten minutes in warm mineral oil, corn oil, or olive oil.
And another: buff the nails with short quick strokes,
always in the same direction.

. . . All hands need a weekly manicure. If you manicure
your own nails, follow these basic steps:

1. Remove old polish with an oily polish remover.
Moisten cotton with the remover and press the
cotton against the nail for several seconds, then pull
the cotton straight up the nail and off. Don't rub
back and forth or in circles. Rinse the nails with
lukewarm water.

2. Never cut the cuticle; it will only grow back
stronger and more ragged. Apply cuticle remover
(using an orange stick tipped with cotton) and push
back the cuticle very gently, working around the
base and sides of the nail and under the tip. Some
brands of cuticle remover work more quickly than
others. Check the instructions on the one you are
using. After specified time, wash it off with warm
soapy water. Dry the hands with a soft towel and
gently rub away the dead cuticle.

3. Shape your nails with an emery board. Don't file too deep at the corners, as this may cause splitting. A rounded oval or slightly squared top is best. Always file in *one* direction, not with a back and forth sawing motion. Use the coarse side of the emery board to shape your nails, the finer side to smooth the edges.

4. With hand steadied on table top, brush on base coat. Allow to dry.

5. Apply polish. The first coat should be thin, the second coat slightly heavier. A light-toned frosted polish may require three coats. In each application, remove a hairline of polish from the tip of each nail. Allow ten minutes between applications of each coat if you can. If that isn't possible, at least be sure each coat is completely dry before the next is brushed on.

. . . Fashions in nails, as with clothes, come and go. It's fun to indulge in some fads occasionally, but do keep within the bounds of attractiveness. Before you go in for eccentric colors and overlong, clawlike nails, be sure your hands lend themselves to such extremes—and that they suit both the occasion *and* your audience.

Some people "frown" with their hands, even when their lips are smiling. Their hands are tight, tense, the veins stand out. For calm looking hands, hold them over your head for a moment or just bend your elbows so that the hands are upright. Then rest your hands in your lap, palms up, one gently resting on the other, and make a conscious effort to keep them relaxed.

Here are some exercises for graceful, flexible hands. Repeat each several times.

For Limbering

1. Make a fist, throw out fingers vigorously, fingers wide apart.

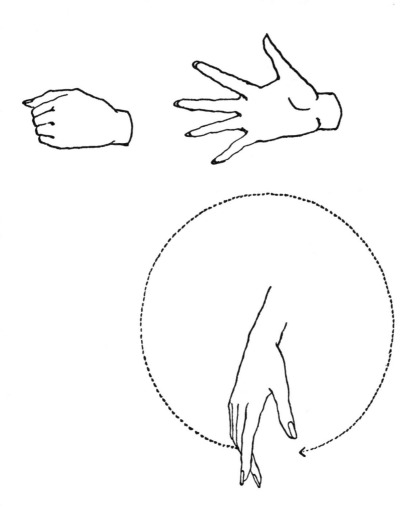

2. Circle hands from wrist in both directions.

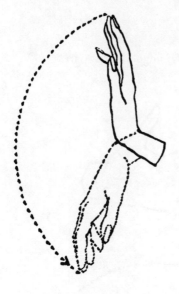

Graceful Movements

1. Lift hand up and down from wrist, keeping hand itself relaxed.

2. Move hands and arms slowly in front of you, in and out. With inward movement, palm is leading; moving outward, wrist leads. Fingers are relaxed and passive.

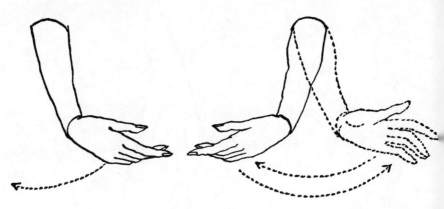

When you are proud of your hands, you'll use them more beautifully. But don't use them to excess. "Talking" with the hands looks affected, nervous, or gauche—so avoid unnecessary gesticulation!

LEGS—THE LONG AND THE SHORT OF IT

A man who seems to specialize in watching legs (and who, incidentally, is an eminent physician in New York) told me that, in the entire history of mankind, legs have never been in better shape. It's all because of better nutrition during formative years, the decline of rickets, and early correction of possible problems. Most of the things that go wrong with legs, he went on to tell me, occur after maturity and are entirely the fault of the owner. Well, let's take a long look at legs—sexy, kicky, sometimes tired-out legs—to see how they can be kept sexy and steadfast.

The fact that basic shapes are better than ever is little consolation if you are one of the not-so-shapelies. You can't make a pair of long, lean stems out of short squat ones, true. However, you can do the best with what you've got and sometimes improve upon nature. Exercise for leg-shaping must be consistent—daily, now and forever. Nine women out of ten have flabby or overlarge thighs by the time they are thirty-five. It's a problem area and only regular exercises plus weight control can prevent, correct, and maintain. Along with daily calisthenics, you can give your legs good exercise and firm the leg muscles evenly by varying your shoe heels. Each heel height exercises muscles that the others don't. Go barefoot sometimes, wear flats for relaxing, low heels for long hikes, medium heels for every day, higher heels for dress-up occasions and your variety will spice your fashion and shape your legs.

Legs are, by nature, rather dry. In most bodies there just aren't enough active oil glands in the limbs to keep them smooth-textured. Use a lubricating lotion often and stroke it on with a strong massaging action, firmly kneading the thigh area.

Even more unfortunate—legs, by nature, grow hair. The word is—off! Depilation—hair removal—should be done as often as needed. Shaving is the fastest method, and although it does not make the hair grow faster or thicker, it does grow in stubbly and may appear heavier. The best method of depilation is waxing, which is generally done in a salon. The most convenient solution for most women is a depilatory used at home. Since depilatories differ in strength and purpose, choose one especially created for removing *leg* hair. Explicit directions are always printed on the container or included in the package. Be sure to follow them carefully. As this type of product works deep in the follicle to melt hair away below the surface, the results are longer-lasting than with shaving.

The *bête-noir* of legs—too-visible veins. If it's the serious problem of varicose veins, go to your doctor who will prescribe treatment or corrective surgery. Often it's a surface condition—little webs of veins that pose no medical problem but look unattractive. Like wrinkles and other flaws, early precaution and prevention is the best course. Avoid impairment of circulation: too-tight girdles, garters, boots, habitual crossing of the legs when seated. Avoid extreme heat: putting your legs too close to the radiator or fireplace, or under-seat heater in train or car, prolonged sunbathing, too-hot baths. Do encourage good circulation by exercising daily, walking daily, by varying your position. Don't sit too long, stand too long, lie too long. An excellent preventive exercise for visible leg veins is the bicycle exercise. You can do it mornings before you arise, evenings before slumber, in the comfort of your bed. Start flat on your back and raise your legs and spine until your weight is resting on your shoulders. Support your back with your hands. Now let your legs pedal like mad for several minutes.

After a long day on your feet, when you get home stretch out with feet raised on pillows. Or lie on the floor with your bare feet, knees up, close as possible to an uncluttered wall. Try to "walk" up the wall. As you go higher, support your back with your hands. When you reach the highest point, hold your feet there for three to five minutes. If you have a tendency to visible leg veins, place a wedge at the bottom of your mattress to raise your feet while you're sleeping.

If broken veins in your leg are embarrassingly evident, don't show them off through sheer hose. You can find textured, patterned, or opaque styles that are quite fashionable. You may want to cover up with a caftan after your swim at beach or pool. Some smaller areas of spidery broken veins can be camouflaged with the makeup you use for concealing under-eye shadows or other facial flaws.

FEET—TEN TINY TOES

The little things that carry you around all day are certainly put upon and too often ill-rewarded. Pretty feet, as the man in the museum pointed out, can be quite exciting. Neglected feet are unattractive and uncomfortable, too. If they are seen, and they often are in open-toed shoes and sandals, they detract from your appearance. If they hurt, your walk suffers—your posture collapses—your very expression and disposition may be affected. If your feet give you problems, check your shoes. Maybe you need another style, a larger size. Throw out (or give away) any pair that hurts. Wearing them is false economy. And watch your hose; too-tight socks or stockings do almost as much harm as too-small shoes.

Here are some tips for foot care
When you bathe, after a long soak, rub any calluses or hard spots with a pumice stone. Scrub your feet thoroughly with a stiff bristle brush, toe by toe, front, arch, sole, and heel. Dry your feet thoroughly—don't skip between the toes—and push back the cuticle on the toenails just as you would your fingernails. Massage your feet with a rich hand or body lotion, working it around each toe, into cuticles, rubbing it well into the heels.

If you are a devotée of the shower, have a foot bath at least twice weekly. Add a little bath oil, bubble bath, milk bath—or soaking salts if your feet are tired—and let them soak for five or ten minutes.

Give yourself a pedicure weekly—use cuticle remover, following the same instructions as for fingernails. Always trim toenails straight across; curving them could encourage ingrown nails.

At the first sign of ingrown nails, corns, calluses, warts, or other blemishes, see a podiatrist.

In summertime—in fact, anytime—dust your feet with a good foot powder, especially between the toes, before you put on your hose. Sprinkle a little foot powder, or talcum powder, inside your shoes.

Give your feet the air. When feet are imprisoned all day—especially in boots that shut off oxygen and build up heat—they can suffer irritation, and even fungus can result. Don't leave your boots on all day if you can help it. Air your feet whenever you can, with open sandals or other unconfining styles. Don't wear the same shoes day after day. Change off for the comfort and health of your feet. Your shoes will last longer, too.

Don't burden your feet. What carries around the excess poundage of the body? The feet, of course. They were created, in length and width, to bear your *normal* weight. Every ounce over puts *them* in bad shape, as well as you.

Exercise your feet. Many foot exercises can be done while you sit reading, talking on the phone, or watching television. Do these with bare feet—each six to ten times:

1. Roll a bottle (small soft drink size) under your bare foot. Start with it under the metatarsal arch. Roll it forward to the toes, then back to the arch.
2. Hold your feet up and try to spread out the toes, as you would spread your fingers. Now wiggle the toes.
3. Put feet flat on the floor. Raise the toes only, while keeping balls of feet on floor. Repeat ten times.

4. Feet flat and parallel, roll each foot to the outer side, curling toes under. Hold for a moment, then return.
5. Put a telephone book under your feet and try to lift the pages with your toes. Or put a small object on the floor (a pencil, matchbook, marble) and try to pick it up with your toes.

THE ALL-IMPORTANTS

The type of deodorant you use depends upon individual need and preference. Best for most women is an antiperspirant deodorant, which serves the dual purpose of eliminating unpleasant odor and keeping the underarms dry. Never apply an antiperspirant immediately after shaving or removing underarm hair by depilation. Let twenty-four hours elapse to avoid the possibility of any irritation. If your hands are inclined to dampness, give them a quick spray of antiperspirant deodorant just before that big dance or the reception where you will be shaking many hands.

A danger spot that may offend—when you're least aware of doing so—is the mouth. Brush your teeth morning and night and after every meal when you can. Use dental floss to remove any food particles that get trapped between the teeth. Beautiful teeth are an asset to every woman. Don't think you can hide the uneven one by not laughing. Don't fool yourself into thinking no one notices that one little gap because it's so far back. Any dental flaw is all too apparent to others. Dentists can work positive magic in capping, restoring, even reshaping. Whatever the investment, consider whether you can afford *not* to make it.

If teeth, gums, and digestion are in perfect order, and if you have been dining on rose petals and nectar, your breath will probably be sweet, or at least acceptable. But why take chances? It's so easy to use a mouthwash—the liquid kind at home, the quick spray when you're away from home. If you love your friends, do avoid eating raw onions, strong-smelling cheese, food with more than a trace of garlic. And remember—parsley is a natural breath freshener. Don't leave it on your plate as a garnish. Eat it! It contains vitamins and iron, too.

What's the most forgotten part of the body? The ears! Although we all too often neglect them or take them for granted, in some cultures ears are considered so sexy that they are kept covered from the eyes of all but one's husband! If your ears are pretty little shells, by all means show them. If they are not pretty, wear your hair in a style that covers at least part of them. In Japan, women include their ears in their face treatment, and it's not a bad idea—especially when the skin is dry. All ears will respond to a touch of moisturizing emulsion smoothed on the external area after their daily cleaning. If your ears *are* attractive, try the faintest touch of blush on the lobes.

And choose your earrings not only to harmonize with your fashion but also to complement the size and shape of your ears.

BATHING FOR BEAUTY

Can you think of a great beauty who wasn't famous—among other things—for her enjoyment of the bath?

They tell us that slaves scoured the hills of ancient Greece for the most fragrant flowers to float in the bath of Helen. Cleopatra, ever sensuous, ever artful, spent hours being anointed with precious oils after her ritual ablution. According to legend, Poppea, the bride of Emperor Nero, owed her satiny skin to daily milk baths and a herd of five hundred she-asses was kept for this express purpose. We've heard of the famous actresses who were up to their necks in champagne—and the not-so-extravagant who soaked in bubbles of another kind. From earliest times right through to the present (with a possible lapse in Europe in the Dark Ages!) the bath has been a tradition and ritual of beauty.

Now the sybaritic bath has caught up with the Space Age. Women are busier than ever; their lives are more filled with tension and anxiety. The shower is quick and efficient. It's great for morning refreshment. However, it doesn't quite take the place of a luxurious bath—one that serves a beauty purpose while it works restorative magic for body and spirit. No matter how many quick splashes and functional dunks are taken for daily cleansing, I strongly recommend that every woman treat herself to a luxurious bath at least once a week.

Since serenity is an integral part of charm, the bath should be an exercise in relaxation as well as a beauty treatment for the entire body. When you take your ritual bath, make it a *beauty* bath. Plan it as carefully as the world's loveliest women did (and do)—and think of it as one of your most deserved luxuries of the day. . . .

First—tie up your hair with a ribbon or protect it with a pretty scarf or bonnet. Thoroughly cleanse your face and throat, following the procedure recommended for your skin type. Now, smooth on a rich lubricating cream. The warmth of the atmosphere will help accelerate its action on your skin. If your skin is oily, you will not use a lubricant, of course, but do "fingerprint" eye cream around the eye area and smooth a refining mask over the rest of your face.

The water for your tub should be just comfortably warm. While your tub is filling, add a bath product that will fill the room with fragrance, scent your skin, and make it lovely to the touch. Today's bounty in bath products are more delightfully fragrant and effective in their purpose beyond the dreams of history's most pampered empress. If your skin feels thirsty all over, choose an aromatic bath oil that will disperse in warm water to reach every dry skin area as you bathe. Or use a bubbling milk bath that will produce mounds of foam to luxuriate in, while its ingredients help silken the skin.

After you have lowered yourself into the tub, place cotton pads, presoaked with cooling herbal extracts, over your eyes to banish any feeling of strain, to help reduce any puffiness, as you relax. Try to release all tension. Think of nothing—or the sublime. After ten or fifteen minutes, when you have completely unwound and the day's cares have vanished, remove the eye pads and stretch your entire body. Think of each part as you stretch it—ankles, legs, thighs, hips, waist, diaphragm, back, chest, shoulders, arms, hands, fingertips. Now lather your washcloth with the finest soap and make long stretching movements, to help posture and waistline, as you wash. Do some of your hand and foot exercises too—or even a few facial gymnastics. After rinsing off the lather, take the pumice stone you should always keep at the side of the tub and gently rub any hard, rough skin on feet, heels, elbows.

Emerge from the tub slowly—like Venus from the sea—and stretch again from head to toe as you pat yourself dry with a fluffy towel. With a tissue, blot from your face and neck any film of lubricating cream remaining on the surface of the skin (most of it will have been absorbed by this time) and get ready for your body complexion treatment. For this you will need a body cream or lotion that is quickly absorbed yet rich in humectants to smooth away dryness and keep the body skin young to the touch and the eye. Take a little lotion in the palm of one hand, then distribute it over both hands. Now, using an upward massage motion, with one hand following the other in light, lifting strokes, smooth the lotion over each leg, over the entire body, back, shoulders, arms. Sit down while you massage it thoroughly into the feet, giving extra attention to dry heels and ankles.

A spray of delightful cologne or toilet water and a fluff of dusting powder will follow. And now—smooth and fragrant to your toe tips and refreshed and serene—you are ready, depending on the hour, for a lovely day, a delightful evening, or to dream beautiful dreams.

6

Fragrance—Your Personal Expression

It's silent. It's invisible. Yet it can say a great deal about you. It's a dimension of your charm, an expression of your personality.

DELIGHT IN VARIETY

You may have a special favorite or lean to fragrances of a similar base. Most women do. You'll keep coming back to that one again and again. Keep it on your perfume tray, of course, but don't overlook the spice a change of fragrance can add to your life. I like to vary the fragrances I wear with the seasons. Spring—a light-hearted scent. Summer— floral notes. Autumn—something zesty and spirited. Winter—a richer, sophisticated scent. Fragrance should be suited to the occasion, too, and even the hour. A heady perfume that might be glamorous at night would be out of place for a morning business meeting. And the crisp, fresh scent so right for morning may be lost on the midnight air. Have enough varieties at hand so that you're always appropriately "dressed" in fragrance, whatever the hour, the occasion, or your mood!

HOW TO CHOOSE FRAGRANCE

When you're shopping for a new fragrance, test only

two at a time. Otherwise, your sense of smell will become confused. The best method is to spray or touch the perfume or cologne to the inside of one clean wrist. By clean I mean free from other scent or lotion; if you had applied anything else to that spot even hours before, it can subtly change the scent you're testing. Wait a moment for the alcohol content to evaporate, then sniff. What you'll notice is the top note. But don't decide yet. Walk around the store for ten minutes, then sniff your wrist again. Now you'll get the full body of the fragrance, as it is interpreted by your chemistry. Now try the second fragrance on the other wrist and repeat the process. When you decide which one lifts your spirits—and expresses *your* personality—go ahead and buy!

HOW TO USE FRAGRANCE

COLOGNE. Spray or smooth cologne (or toilet water, which is just a little stronger) all over the body after bath or shower.

DUSTING POWDER. Follows the cologne with powder. If your body skin is dry, skip the dusting powder, especially in winter.

PERFUME. More intense in fragrance than either cologne or toilet water, perfume should be touched to the skin at strategic spots: wrists, inside elbows, around the ears, in the hollow of the throat, decolletage, behind the knees.

Never apply perfume or cologne to fabric or fur. The essential oils and alcohol in these products can possibly stain or weaken fabric. If you *must,* limit the spraying or dabbing to a handkerchief, the inner band of a hat, the back of a lapel or even the back of a label.

A spray of cologne on your hair is a charming touch, especially if you'll be dancing all night with a tall partner. However, since it is drying to delicate hair strands, save this for very special evenings.

When it's a sizzling day and the air conditioner isn't

working, try this "quick cooler" with fragrance. Saturate a big wad of cotton with a light-scented eau de cologne. Run the wad of fragrant cotton up one arm, around the back of the neck, down the other arm, across your midriff (if it's bare), behind your knees. This is a wonderful quick-cleanser too, if you're on a camping trip or otherwise far from civilization.

HOW OFTEN TO APPLY

Some people seem to carry fragrance with them wherever they go. In fact, they're known as "perfume carriers." It's generally conceded that fragrance is longer-lasting and more pronounced on women who have more natural oils in their skin. I suspect that some of the "perfume carriers" I know also use fragrance more lavishly!

As a rule, a fragrance impression will last three to four hours. Then "touch-up" with a purse size or an extra bottle of cologne or perfume you may keep in your office or your club locker.

Our own olfactory senses become accustomed to a scent after a time. Others may be much more aware of the fragrance you're wearing than you are. Strike a happy balance. Don't overpower your audience, but do wear enough so that you feel wrapped in a pleasant aura. Your fragrance is your personal expression—and *you* should delight in it, too.

7

Hair That Makes Headlines

If newspapers had been part of the medieval scene, can you imagine the headlines Lady Godiva would have created? Riding through town on a snow white horse, with only her flowing blonde hair for a cloak, was sure to make news! While few can surpass her for originality, throughout history women of wisdom and charm have appreciated the value of a good head of hair. And they have been well aware of its magnetic effect on the male. Beautiful hair has always been considered a vital element of sex appeal. It's little wonder, then, that women have been curling, coloring, and caring for their hair since earliest recorded time with the best means available. The "best" was pretty bad for thousands of years. Women suffered inconvenience, sometimes pain, often risk (of losing their hair entirely!) with primitive methods of coaxing their locks to what was considered the high fashion of their day.

Today, women are still curling, coloring, and caring for their hair—but with a wonderful difference. Contemporary methods are simple, effective, and readily available. An empress of long ago might have traded her crown jewels for the treasury of hair products the average modern woman has at her fingertips. Now any woman who will give just a little time and attention to this important part of her appearance can "make headlines" with her tresses.

KNOW YOUR OWN HAIR

Are you aware that hair is almost as individual as fingerprints? In fact, stray strands have been used as evidence not only by detectives but also by wives!

Your hair is a complex cellular structure. Each strand, as skinny and uncomplicated as it may look to the naked eye, consists of several layers. The core (central medulla) is surrounded by the cortex which, in turn, is covered by the outside surface of cuticle. Hair usually grows at the rate of half an inch monthly and each strand will last up to seven years. There are approximately 100,000 strands of hair on the average head, and it is quite normal for a few old ones to be sloughed off daily as new strands take their place.

Never forget that your hair is a living part of your body, nourished by the bloodstream (that's how the vitamins in the food you eat get to deposit strength and gleam in the strands), and lubricated by the oil glands in the scalp.

Hair that has bounce, shine, a look of vitality, is the result of a good working body teamed with a program of correct care. Some hair looks "old" (just as some complexions do) long before it should. A dull, lifeless look, dandruff, imbalance of oils, and other problems may stem from illness, diet deficiency, lack of sleep, too many self-prescribed pills, a buildup of tension, or even emotional upset. When hair is *really* sick—falling out in handfuls or badly flaked with dandruff, and when it doesn't respond to external treatment—something's wrong inside. Consult your doctor.

The natural color of your hair, its texture, and whether it is straight or curly is determined by the genes. So is the tendency to strong or weak hair. If you're not satisfied with the inherited characteristics, you can't change your great-grandparents. However, the know-how of keeping your hair in gleaming condition, shimmering with attractive color, and fashionably styled, can make up for many of nature's shortcomings.

Take an analytical look at your hair from time to time and give it the touch test. The inherent structure doesn't change, but everything else about it is subject to internal and external influences. Is your knowledge of your own hair *au courant?* What is its texture: fine, medium, or coarse? What is its density: thin, average, or thick? What is its condition: dry, normal, oily, or combination (oily at roots, dry along strands)? What is the degree of curliness? How does it react to seasonal changes, to humidity, to chemicals? Is the color even, is it attractive, is it in harmony with skintone and personality? Is your hair healthy—smooth and silken to the very ends? Once you really know your hair you can proceed with confidence to find the best plan for its care.

THE "ALL-IMPORTANTS" FOR PRETTY HAIR

Style and color may draw raves—but they won't mean a thing unless your hair is enjoying good health. Here are some building blocks on which to base hair beauty:

THE FUNDAMENTALS

First on the list is a well-balanced diet, with enough vitamins (vitamin A is especially important for good hair) and minerals. Get sufficient sleep. And exercise for good circulation—yes, that blood nourishes the scalp, too!

BRUSHING

Daily brushing stimulates the scalp, distributes oils from the scalp along the full length of the hair, removes dust and loose strands, and adds glisten and gleam to your whole beautiful mane! A brush with natural bristles is best. Bend forward from the waist—or sit in a chair with the upper part of your body completely dropped over—to bring blood to the scalp for added circulation. Now, starting with the brush close to the scalp, make long, lifting strokes down the entire length of the hair, giving a twist to your brush as you reach the ends. Divide the hair in sections so that you reach every area. If your hair had been teased, brush *tenderly* until all the snarls are out and then proceed with the long, sweeping strokes. Keep a piece of toweling handy and wipe your brush off frequently as you use it. Wash your brush often by swishing the bristles through mild soapsuds. Always dry it with bristles down.

MASSAGE

To loosen tense muscles in the scalp and to improve circulation, massage your scalp before every shampoo—or whenever you have a few private moments (perhaps while you're sitting alone before the TV). Place your hands at the back of your head and, using the complete flat hand—palms as well as fingers—rotate slowly and gently. Move the hands up the sides of the head, the crown, the front, continuing the rotating action. Be sure the *scalp* is moving, not just your hands. Don't dig in or rub briskly. The word is gentle and the tempo is slow.

DON'T ABUSE

Hair can't scream and it doesn't transmit pain. But it has its own way of "crying" when it's hurt. The ends split, the strands become brittle and lackluster. What hurts hair? Overexposure to sun, for one thing. Hair gets sunburned, just as your skin does. Protect it from strongest rays with a hat or scarf, especially if your hair is dry or tinted. Chemicals can hurt, too. If you use tints, bleaches, permanents, straighteners, or sprays, be sure to counterbalance with correct conditioning. Swimmers should be aware that chlorinated pool water can damage hair and fade the color of tinted hair. Wear a swim cap, of course, and be sure to rinse your hair thoroughly in clear water and then use conditioner, after your swim. Also abusing are tension or friction. Hair pulled back too tightly into a ponytail or knot can induce a receding hairline. Daily use of brush rollers, especially if you sleep on them or if they are pulled so tightly that the brush presses on your scalp, can cause scalp irritation. Using heated rollers too consistently, without benefit of conditioners, or using the hottest setting on your hair dryer can dehydrate your hair and lead to breakage.

SHAMPOO FOR SHINE!

Beautiful hair is immaculately clean hair, gleaming with lovely highlights. Your regular shampoo is the primary step in hair care and should never be run through haphazardly. Follow these simple steps to make it a delightful beauty ritual:

• First, brush your hair thoroughly and massage the scalp for two or three minutes.
• Wet hair with warm water.
• Apply shampoo, working it through the hair and scalp with massaging action.
• Rotate the fingertips in small circles, but don't dig in with your fingernails! Rinse thoroughly with warm running water. (A spray attachment on your faucet is a big help.)
• If hair is normal, oily, or heavily coated with spray, repeat the application of shampoo for a second lathering. If hair is dry or brittle, use only one lathering.
• After the final lathering, rinse, rinse, rinse. Be sure every last soap bubble has been washed away from the scalp, hairline, and every strand of hair. Even the slightest residue of soap will leave a dulling film. When you're sure your hair has been rinsed "squeaking clean," use cold water for the "grand finale" stimulating rinse.
• Wrap your head in a towel and blot dry. Vicious rubbing is not necessary and can damage sensitive hair.

How often to shampoo?

NORMAL TO DRY HAIR. Once a week is average. However, if your hair is exposed to dust, to pollution-laden city air, to smoke, or other besmirchers, wash it more often. Use a mild shampoo and follow with conditioner.

OILY HAIR. At least twice a week or as often as needed. Use a shampoo especially formulated to control and improve the balance of lubrication.

BRITTLE, SUPERSENSITIVE, OR ABUSED HAIR. Shampoo once a week. Use a gentle shampoo followed by a rich conditioner. If hair is badly abused, use a deep conditioner instead of shampoo on alternate weeks until you see definite improvement.

FOR PERFECTION CONDITION

Regular conditioning is a protective for all hair; it's a "must" for any hair that shows signs of dryness and dullness, or that has been tinted, dyed, permanented, or straightened. There are various types of conditioners available, and the one you use should be carefully selected for your specific need.

DEEP CONDITIONING. This is essential for hair that is extremely dry, that has been abused or damaged. Deep conditioners come in cream or oil form, to be applied after the shampoo and left in the hair for ten, fifteen, or twenty minutes to allow the rich ingredients to penetrate the hair shaft. If hair is in very bad condition, a weekly deep conditioning is recommended until there is definite improvement. Then deep condition on alternate weeks until perfection is reached. For all hair (except oily) a monthly deep conditioning treatment is a good "tonic." If your hair is oily, but the ends are dry, apply deep conditioner to the dry ends only.

INSTANT CONDITIONING. Accomplish with a liquid (generally containing protein) that is combed through freshly washed, towel-dried hair. The instant conditioner adds strength and bounce to the hair and also serves as a setting lotion. It's easy to use, fast and efficient for all hair—gives body to fine hair.

CREAM RINSE. Use after your shampoo to untangle snarls and leave hair beautifully soft and lustrous. It's recommended for normal and dry hair. However, if your hair is very fine and thin, a cream rinse may leave it so soft that it doesn't hold a set and becomes a little hard to keep in line.

HAIR STYLING FOR INDIVIDUALITY

The way you wear your hair is a banner headline that announces to the world your personality, your individual fashion, and your relation to current trends. Throughout history coiffures have reflected the temper of their times, at various points expressing romance, arrogance, conformity, and even rebellion!

In very recent memory women were obedient to the arbiters of hair fashion and insistent on having their hair dressed in the "latest style" whatever it may have been at the time and whether or not it was personally becoming. I recall the passing parade of wind-blowns, poodle cuts, artichokes, bouffants—each in its day so universally popular it became a sort of uniform for the head. At this moment, however, there is great freedom of expression. Young women, especially, are completely uninterested in serving as showcases for a hairdresser's latest design; they prefer to wear their hair in delightfully natural ways that display its own beauty—its swing, its color, and its texture. Even women whose weekly salon visits are a "must" are choosing styles that are less contrived, less stereotyped, and far more suited to their features and their personal needs. Style, at least for the moment, has been put in its place—where it relates rather than overpowers.

Some women enjoy changing their coiffures as often as their skirt lengths. Others adopt a style they enjoy and it becomes a long-term acquisition. When I first arrived in the United States from Paris, I wore my hair in a short cut *à la garcon*. It was fashionable, yet very easy to maintain. Later, when I was traveling almost continuously on a tight time schedule, I wanted a completely different style, but one with built-in advantages. I had to have a coiffure that would look well-groomed from morning till night; one that would not be blown apart at the airport just before I was to face a TV camera or collapse in humidity as I was about to start my business schedule. I found that long hair drawn into a chignon at the back of my head was the answer. These many years later, I am wearing my hair in essentially the same way. In keeping with passing trends, from time to time the chignon has moved higher or lower and the crown of my coiffure has risen an inch or gone flatter. However, the basic style hasn't changed. Being human and female, I have had a recurrent urge for a completely different look, but since any mention of cutting brings protests from friends, I have resisted! My need for change is satisfied by letting my hair fall free on leisurely weekends or on quiet evenings at home, or catching it in a ribbon or scarf for most casual occasions.

Every woman should evaluate her hair style at least twice a year. Some coiffures are classic—others become dated. If you have a yen for a new coiffure, study all its possibilities before you adopt it. Fashions in hair styles come and go, but the basic structure of your face is yours forever. Whatever the current vogue, shape the line to frame *your* face shape. The following chart will give you general guidance.

SHAPE YOUR HAIR TO YOUR FACE

Every shape face can be interesting. The squareness or roundness, the heart-shape or whatever-shape of yours can give it a piquancy all its own. These suggestions are general and intended for those who prefer to create illusions that, subtly modify the dimensions of one's face in the eye of the beholder.

OVAL FACE

Any number of styles will look wonderful! However, if nature has given you a classically perfect shape, why not show it off with a simple, smooth line?

ROUND FACE

To create an illusion of length, add fulness at the top, rather than the sides. If bangs are desired, keep them high off the forehead. Shorter hair (eartip length) is preferable. Push longer hair behind the ears.

SQUARE FACE

Keep the line soft, with fullness below the ears, to make the face seem less angular. Depending on your age, moderately long to long hair can be attractive. Try a side part, or sweep the hair to one side for an interesting look.

LONG FACE

Part hair on the side and comb it straight across the crown, preferably with curved bangs. Medium length is best, with width at the sides to give the illusion of a shorter face. If hair is longer, be sure it's soft and full below the temples.

HEART-SHAPED FACE

(This face has a wide forehead and a narrow chin line.) An off-center or side part, with bangs curving out at either side, will make the forehead appear narrower. Hair should be closer to the head above the cheeks, fuller and soft below the cheek line.

TRIANGULAR FACE

(This face has a narrow forehead and a wide jaw line.) Hair should be full and fluffy on top and at the temples to create an impression of greater width in the forehead area. Keep hair closer to the head below the temples. Bangs can be attractively softening.

Here are some other points to keep in mind in selecting a new style or in judging whether your present style is the best one for you:

...The style should be right for your face *from every angle;* as attractive from side and back as it is from the front.

... The style must suit your body as well as your head. A full, long hairdo is out of proportion on a small woman. A tall woman can wear longer hair or a fuller coiffure. A long neck will look *too* swanlike when hair is swept high on the head; it looks beautiful with a chignon low on the nape. A short neck disappears into long hair or hair that is full around the neck; an upswept coiffure makes the neck seem longer than it is.

... Consider the texture of your hair. Thin, fine hair doesn't lend itself to a shoulder-length style, it will separate and droop. Curly hair is more manageable when it's short. Gleaming hair, rich in color, deserves to be shown off in a silken sweep with smooth lines that catch the light.

... Your age, your personality, your activities should influence your choice of style. If you're under twenty, the more natural the better. An active sportswoman should choose a simple, easily handled coiffure. A career woman wants to combine chic with efficiency. A model, actress, or social butterfly can indulge in a greater variety of styles that require more time and attention. The mature woman should avoid long, straight hair styles because they accent any downward trend of the contour; she'll find softness around the face and hair length just below the eartips more appealing. A stylized coiffure can be interesting on an elegant woman. "Chi-chi" styles look glamorous after dark but are as inappropriate as a ball gown for day.

. . . Most important of all, the basis of an attractive, well-mannered hair style is an expert *cut.* There's a fine art to shaping hair and it should be left to one who has expert "know-how."

YOUR CROWNING COLOR

Whether natural or acquired, the color of your hair plays a starring role in your total look, and the rest of your color scheme revolves around it. It is reflected in your skintone. It determines your choice of makeup shades. It blends or contrasts with your fashion colors, resulting in either harmony or discord. As a vital part of your self-identity, it sways many a mood and action.

Hair of a ravishing color is one of Nature's most generous gifts. If you are among the fortunate, don't tamper with your natural tone. Just pamper your tresses and keep them healthily bright, the better to display their lovely lights. However, if nature was not so kind or if your once-beautiful color has faded with time, there's no point in sighing over what might have been when you can plot a colorful future. Today's hair color cosmetics can change drab to dazzling, give a lift to your looks, and another dimension to your life. You can add a few highlights without changing the basic tone. You can go a few degrees lighter or darker or move all the way to a completely new color. You can cover gray or tone it to scrumptious silver. When one's dream shade may be achieved so easily, few women can resist the temptation—and few do!

Some years ago, when I would hear that plaintive query, "Miss Rubinstein, do you think I should color my gray hair?" I would often answer, "No, it's lovely as it is." Now I feel and speak differently. Any woman who has reached the point of *asking* has already given the subject considerable thought. She's dissatisfied with the status quo. Others may look at her gray hair and say, "Beautiful." She gazes in the mirror and says, "Age." Changing from gray to a soft, youthful shade has given many women a new lease on life.

Some women in their thirties find their hair color is fading. There may not be any gray strands, but often there is a dulling of the tone that gives a nondescript look. A pickup of color helps to freshen the entire personality—and helps a woman of thirty-five or more to look as young as she feels. I recommend it!

On the other hand, however, I don't encourage young girls to change their natural hair tone. Any shade, when the hair is healthily vital, can be beautiful. The right makeup and costume colors and a shampoo that highlights the natural shade are sometimes all that is needed to bring the natural tone out of the shadows and into the spotlight. The quality, texture, and tone of natural hair can never be surpassed by chemically induced color.

There are exceptions when the need is psychological as well as physical. I know a young woman who had experienced a number of problems and who seemed "beaten down" by life by the time she was twenty-three. She attributed her inferiority complex to her nose, which was not perfect though I felt it was not out of proportion to her face. She came to me with a plea that I recommend a plastic surgeon. I prevailed upon her to delay that drastic step. "First become a blonde," I suggested. "It's much less expensive and will do more for you." She agreed half heartedly, and I instructed the hairstylist not to let her look in a mirror until the process was completed, her hair combed, and until a makeup artist had created a new "sunny face" to go with her new hair. The result was dramatic. From the moment she saw her transformed self in the mirror, she seemed to take on a new personality. She looked different and she decided to make a different life for herself. She bought a wardrobe of more colorful, more feminine clothes. She put brighter touches into her apartment. She started to meet new people. I know you expect me to tell you she married her dream man. Actually, she broke her long-standing engagement to a rather dull fellow, and when I last saw her the big excitement of her life was the boutique she had just opened. This was her choice, and I was impressed by the fact that she was planning her life and living it fully—not being pushed by circumstances.

A complete change in hair color can be a big step for many women. Sometimes it is warranted, sometimes not. This is something every woman should consider carefully—and perhaps seek qualified advice on—before taking the plunge. Of course, every change need not be drastic. There are many degrees of change and various methods for different needs and effects.

Temporary color rinse

If you want a small "lift" of color, try a temporary color rinse first. It coats the hair with color, without penetrating the shaft to affect your actual tone. You can add highlights of red or blond, intensify your own color, or deepen your own shade. However, you can't go lighter in color with a temporary rinse, and you can't cover gray (though you may be able to blend in a few scattered gray hairs). The rinse washes out when you shampoo (some brands last through several shampoos) so that you can easily cancel out any mistake. This is the easiest to use and the easiest on your hair, but provides very limited scope for color change.

Permanent tint

This assures more definite change. You can go darker or you can go lighter to a limited degree—one or two tones for most hair. You can cover gray completely. Since a permanent tint will last until the hair grows out, choose your new shade with care and be sure it will complement your skintone. Generally speaking, a shade just a little lighter than your own natural hair color is best. Tinted hair that is darker than your natural color may have a harsh look. Permanent tints are mixed with a special peroxide and used according to the specific directions enclosed in the package. Generally, the first application is to the entire length of hair and all subsequent applications (retouches) are to new root growth only.

Bleach and tone
This is the two-step process that is necessary for a drastic change from a darker to a lighter shade—black to light brown, brunette to blonde, or brownette to redhead, for example. It involves stripping the pigment from the hair by bleaching. The darker your hair is to start with, and the lighter in tone you want to go, the more bleaching will be required. The second step is to add an attractive tone to the bleached-out hair. Understandably, the chemical action on the hair can be quite harsh and a broad change (dark brunette to light blonde, for example) should be weighed carefully. Unless your hair is very strong, it would be advisable to plan a less revolutionary revision.

Streaking and highlighting
Some of the most attractive color effects are achieved by bleaching or coloring selected strands of hair and leaving the rest unchanged. The look can be surprisingly natural or quite dramatic, depending on the amount of hair changed and your color choice. Streaking is a popular technique for an interesting look without a total color change, and it's a great way to blend in a scattering of gray. On blonde or brown hair, highlighting or frosting—with the topmost hair lighter and brighter—gives an appealing sunlit look. The possibilities are many. An expert colorist will sometimes use several shades of tint on one head, blending tones from lighter at the front and side to gradually darker in the back. One of the advantages of streaking and highlighting is that there's not such a marked "grow-in" as with hair

that has been totally colored. Some women can let several months elapse between appointments with their colorists.

When your mind is set, think twice before you decide it's a do-it-yourself job. Some women are adept at such things. Others prefer to have it done at the beauty salon. If you plan to make the color change yourself, check in advance on the procedure. Be sure you get good advice on the product to use and on shade selection. Read all the directions with infinite care before you start and follow step by step. Don't forget to protect your hands against staining by wearing rubber gloves—and use a plastic cape over your shoulders.

Things to remember when you change your hair color

. . . Hair grows at the rate of about half an inch a month—which means roots will be contrasting blatantly if you don't touch up every four weeks.

. . . Whenever you wash your hair, use a gentle shampoo that won't strip color from your tinted hair.

. . . Permanent tints, bleaching, and lightening generally have a drying effect. Regular conditioning is *most* important.

. . . Don't expose your hair to strong sun. Sun can fade, streak, and redden your chemical color. Wear a scarf or hat at the beach or stay in the shade. Be sure to wear your bathing cap when you swim, especially in chlorine-treated water.

. . . When Nature planned your color scheme, she gave you hair, complexion, eyes, eyebrows, and lashes that "go together" in perfect harmony. Since changing your hair color can disturb the natural harmony, you must bring it *all* in tune with the right makeup. Brunettes who have turned blonde often need a slightly warmer shade of foundation and makeup, with lipstick and cheek color on the peachy side. If you've gone darker you may need subtler tones. Adding red to the hair can make the skin look sallow; a makeup foundation with pink or peach tones to brighten the complexion will make you look more like a born redhead. In every case, watch your eyebrows and blend both eyebrow makeup and lashes with your new hair shade. Let your mirror be your guide and if you're in doubt, seek the help of a makeup artist. It's worth the effort to assure all harmony and no sour notes in your total color symphony!

To curl

Permanents give body to thin, lank hair that needs more fullness. And, of course, they give curly tops to those with naturally straight hair. If you can manage without a permanent, so much the better for your hair. If your hair *does* need a permanent, be surre it is good condition before you start. Use a deep, rich conditioner one week before your permanent and again the week after. If you tint or bleach, schedule your permanent at the middle of your retouch cycle—at least two weeks after hair coloring and at least two weeks before your next processing. A permanent over a permanent can damage the hair. Be sure all the hair previously permanented has been clipped off. If you want to get best results, don't have a permanent when you're not feeling well. A bad cold, a virus, a migraine headache, even medication in your system can ruin your permanent. Either your hair won't take well, or it may not take at all.

Or uncurl

While straight-haired lasses are trying to encourage curl, those who have it seem determined to iron it out! I don't know why. Curly hair can be very pretty and before you give it up do try a new, more manageable style. Short hair is generally best and displays the natural curl to good advantage. A cream rinse after shampoo will make curly hair easier to manage. Use a firm holding setting lotion and large rollers if you want to induce a smoother line. Straightening of the hair requires some rather strong chemicals and should be left to a professional. Straightened hair is sensitive and requires the most tender care, with regular conditioning.

HOW TO CHOOSE A HAIRSTYLIST

In a word, *carefully!* A good deal about the way you look (and feel about yourself) depends on the person who cuts, colors, styles your hair. So it's worth taking a little time to find the right one.

If you like the way a friend's hair looks, ask her for the name of her stylist. Ask a stranger, for that matter, if you're really impressed. Be aware, however, that the stylist who does fantastic things with your friend's curly top may not have a talent for giving your fine, straight hair the look you want. However, a recommendation is surely a good start.

If you don't have a recommended operator when you make your salon appointment, do give the receptionist a few clues as to what you want. For example: "I'm into sports and want a style I needn't fuss with between appointments"; "I want a cut to make the most of my hair's natural curl"; "Can you give me a colorist who's good with fragile hair?" In every salon, there are operators who have special talents in particular areas. When the receptionist knows your special need, she'll be better able to assign the operator to please you.

When the operator is truly right for you, there'll be good communication. Make clear what you want in style or color or ask for suggestions. You should be able to discuss any problems you may have with your hair and feel that the operator is attentive and interested in helping to find the solution. Don't be shy about speaking up if things are not progressing to your satisfaction—if too much hair is being clipped off, for example, or if you're uncomfortable for any reason. It's your hair and your money.

If you're not thoroughly pleased after your first appointment, ask for another operator next time. If the next one doesn't satisfy either, try another salon. If you've been using the same operator for years, but feel a change is advisable, you might take the timid way out and switch your appointment to your present stylist's day off.

A hair stylist you see regularly knows that your patronage is based on satisfaction and generally will be sincere in suggesting extra services—a body wave, a course of conditioning treatments, a color change. However, don't be intimidated into following any suggestion if you're not totally in accord. Think it over until next time, or just say, "No, thanks." If you're traveling, in a strange town, or for any reason find yourself a one-time-only client, don't be talked into any major or expensive services. Wait and discuss the idea with your regular stylist.

Once you've found a stylist who really knows how to turn your hair into a shining asset, and with whom you have good rapport, treasure him or her! How many *other* people in this world can do so much for your looks and morale in just a couple of hours?

8
A Question of Age

Have you ever had someone stand before you, look you straight in the eye and ask that unanswerable question . . . "How old do you think I am?" I've been asked it many times and have learned it is wise never to give a direct answer. What the woman is asking, of course, is not for a number but for reassurance that she looks ten or fifteen years younger than her calendar age. In any event, I'm the last one in the world to ask because I never think in terms of calendar years. What does it matter? Why should one be tied to a statistic? I believe that birthdays should be celebrated, never deplored, and not necessarily counted.

As the saying goes, how old you are is not as important as *how* you are old. Youth is wonderful. It's a joy to see pretty girls, shiny and saucy and full of promise. Yet, when it comes to true beauty, the honors often go the the woman richer in years whose fashion sense and polished grooming, enthusiasm for life, and charm of manner reflect the wisdom she has acquired through experience.

I can think of a dozen women of "a certain age" (as the French so delicately phrase it) whose faces regularly decorate the pages of newspapers and magazines, whose romances become legend, who fly back and forth on what seems to be a nonstop schedule, who take the spotlight at gala balls, who are sought after by the most eligible men, admired by all. I know many more who may never hit the papers but who, having reached what was once considered "middle age" or even "advanced age," are enjoying it to the hilt.

When meeting any one of these women—the famous or the not-famous—one doesn't think of her years but only that she is an attractive, vital woman. How do they do it? Why do some women seem ageless, magnetic, and beautiful when others with matching dates on their birth certificates seem to be on a headlong downhill ride?

There are a combination of factors. Geneticists place great stress on inherent qualities. It's true that some families retain their good physical condition and a look of youth that belies their years, but they still have to work for it. I've noticed that these families generally have a tradition of sound living. Taking care of one's health—good nutrition, regular exercise, sufficient rest—is a regular investment that pays off later in life. Also of vital importance— mental attitude. We'll talk more about that later. Concern about one's appearance is an extension of mental attitude and part of a happy cycle, since a pleasing reflection in the mirror certainly helps one's frame of mind.

The woman who wants to "grow beautiful" instead of "grow older" has to give *more* attention and more *careful* attention to every facet of her appearance than her younger sister does. A girl may skip her nightly beauty routine or morning exercises occasionally; a woman may *not*. A woman need not spend a great deal of time on her daily beauty program but she must be consistent; she must follow it *every* day without exception. A girl may let her hair blow free and look casual; a woman must guard against looking unkempt when her hair isn't in place. A girl may buy impulsively and wear her mistake; a woman can't live with fashion failures. A woman must be meticulously groomed at every moment, for her own morale as well as her audience's approval. A woman must make beauty a part of her life—but it's worth the effort since in doing so she will discover a new dimension of joy for herself and bring pleasure to those around her.

The guidelines change with the years. The attention a mature woman gives her appearance must be specialized and suited to her now-different needs. Here are some pointers that I have given to women of "a certain age" and "a beautiful age" and which have been applied with great success.

SKIN CARE

The tendency is for complexions to become progressively drier after thirty, and tiny lines become more easily etched in parched skin. Limit the number of soap-and-water washings you give your face and throat. If you *do* use soap, choose the mildest, creamiest kind, and follow each washing with a moisturizing emulsion or lubricant. However, if your skin is truly dry (and especially if it is sensitive) you would be wise to avoid any soaping of your face. Instead, use a light-textured cleansing cream (or cleansing lotion) night and morning and before every makeup change. It will clean deeply without robbing your skin of natural oils and moisture. After you tissue off the cleanser, "rinse" your skin with a gentle freshener. A night cream, rich in emollients, becomes more and more of a necessity with each passing year. Be sure to apply it nightly, or if more convenient, for an hour or so during the day.

Throats, eyes, and hands are the great betrayers of age. The eye area is extremely delicate, practically devoid of natural oil glands, yet subject to greatest impact of expression lines. Use a specially formulated eye cream to keep this vulnerable area gently lubricated. Include your throat in all your facial care and give it the accelerated action of a special throat-firming cream. If you choose one that is nongreasy, you can apply it in the morning, before dressing, as well as at bedtime. Give your hands all the pampering care they need, including a lubricating lotion after every washing.

A word about sunbathing: CAUTION. In recent years

scientists have proved beyond doubt that exposure to bright sunlight is the primary factor in prematurely aging the skin. In addition to parching and dehydrating, it contributes to the uneven coloring, freckling, and blotching that often become evident in middle age. The effects of sunbathing accumulate and, like a time bomb, explode much later on. Unfortunately, the damage can't be reversed. Blondes, redheads, all fair-skinned people are especially susceptible to complexion damage from the sun's rays. They would be wise to hug the shade. And all women who went to keep a fresh, young-looking complexion should avoid the sun at its zenith, limit their sunbathing, and apply an effective sunscreen before every exposure as well as an emollient lotion after every exposure.

MAKEUP

Always apply a moisturizing emulsion to freshly cleansed skin as a prelude to makeup. It helps protect against the elements as it imparts the look and feeling of youthful dewiness. Smooth it over the face and throat. If the skin is especially lacking in moisture, apply a little extra to the parched areas: cheeks, under eyes. After the moisturizing emulsion has been thoroughly absorbed, smooth on a light-textured makeup foundation. One with a cream or oil base is best. A heavy foundation, or one that is too dry, will look harsh and will accent any lines. Use face powder lightly and be sure to brush any excess from lined areas.

Fluff on the subtlest blush of cheek color, keeping it high on the cheekbone and letting it fade off toward the temple. Use a pastel shade of lipstick. Some women tell me their lipstick "bleeds" into the tiny lines around their mouths. To avoid this, when you apply your makeup base smooth it over the lips and pat a little face powder over it. This will form a good foundation for lipstick that stays in place.

Eye makeup is especially important to the mature

woman, as without it eyes can have a faded and expression-less look. However, the entire effect must be subtle, gentle. On the lid itself, shades of pale blue, pale green, or delicate amber are prettiest. If eye shadow is used on the area between lid and brow, a neutral contouring shade may be selected. If the skin is dry or a little loose in this area, use a cream shadow.

Eyebrows should be neatly groomed and lightly accented. Too many mature women overemphasize their brows with too dark a shade or too sharp a line. Check your shade; the color that was perfect for you a few years ago may be too dark now. Apply your eyebrow makeup with tiny, feathery strokes. Avoid the forlorn look that comes when the outside corners of the eyebrows droop. Give the ends a little lift.

When a makeup artist wants to make a youngish woman appear older, for a stage or TV role, one of the first things he does is powder over her lashes. Lashes look young. In fact, they *are* young. It is an unfortunate fact of life that as one grows older lashes become more sparse and less sweeping. Mature women must accent their lashes with mascara (brown, blue, or charcoal shades are prefer-able to black). If your lashes have really done a disappear-ing act, adopt the artificial kind. I don't know of any other makeup item that more effectively subtracts years, adds glamour and attractiveness, all in a minute. Of course, you won't choose a heavy lash as the effect may be too stagy. A natural style in brown or a soft ash shade will give you a whole new lease on beauty.

HAIR

Like your skin, your hair tends to become drier as you grow older. It poses other problems. Often it becomes thinner. Almost invariably it loses its color. Even hair that doesn't turn gray may become drab in tone, lusterless, and tired-looking. There's no doubt about it—with rare excep-tions, hair needs more and more attention as time goes by.

Young girls are hair conscious and work hard to keep their locks shining and beautiful. Mature women too often take the easy way out. Some of them have told me frankly that they prefer a style that's simple to comb rather than one that is twice as attractive but requires a little more handling. The effect is what one would expect: purely utilitarian. Also, too many depend on frequent permanents to solve their hair problems when they should put more emphasis on regular care—daily brushing, scalp, massage, gentle shampoo, and *weekly* conditioning. Unless you have the will to give your hair good care and unless you can develop the knack to do so effectively, keep a steady date with a really good hairdresser.

In choosing your hair style, stay away from straight lines or long-hanging hairdos as these emphasize any downward pull of the contour. Medium length hair, coming just below the eartips, is a good choice. Soft lines, a gentle curl or wave, possibly a slight curve upward at the temple, are generally most flattering. And do avoid, all costs, that frizzy, grizzled overpermanented hair style that screams "middle-aged."

If you have long hair, drawn to the back, you may need the softness of a wave on the sides or a curl at the temple to offset any stark effect. if your hair is lifted up in the back, be sure your rear hairline is worth viewing; with many women this is a spot where hair thins out. If it looks skimpy, keep your chignon low. Very short hair calls attention to the neck and ears. Can yours stand it?

Color makes hair pretty and keeps it looking young. Gray hair that is truly silver or a dramatic salt and pepper can be beautiful. If you're fortunate enough to have it, you may need only a highlighting rinse to win raves. However, most hair doesn't change to a ravishing platinum or fascinating mix. it just becomes mousy, drab, and aging. When it does, it's time to choose a pretty new shade. it's generally best *not* to try to recapture your original color. The identical shade, in artificial color, always looks harsher. You'll find a hair shade just a little lighter actually looks more natural. Many mature women find that lighter tones, especially those that lean to ash rather than reddish hues, are especially flattering. One of the great advantages of having one's hair turn gray is that many blonde shades can be achieved without the long, harsh process of prebleaching. Always a silver lining!

YOUR BODY

Don't you hate that expression "middle-age spread"? Unfortunately, it's more than an expression—it's a reality! The great majority of women over forty tend to be overweight, and too often their excess pounds are in the wrong places. A heavy, poorly toned body is a burden to drag around. In addition, it makes you look older than you are. Why put up with it? Getting back to normal weight may take a lot of discipline, but it's well worth the sacrifice.

Even if your weight is just right today, don't overlook the fact that as the years add up, pounds settle in more easily. The gain can be so gradual that it catches you unaware. The best policy is vigilance. It's far easier to make small sacrifices to hold the line than the greater ones a reducing program demands. To maintain normal weight— and for added vitality—cut down on starches, sweets, fried foods, snacks; concentrate on protein, vegetables, leafy greens, fruits. Find a nutritious diet and let it become *your* Food for Beauty.

How much regular exercise do you give your body? If it's not getting enough, it can become flabby (even without overweight), your circulation may be impaired, and before long you'll find yourself moving with stiff awkwardness. I've seen women in their thirties shambling along as though every step required effort. I've seen women in their eighties move as gracefully as ballerinas. Without exception, those who retain youthful, smooth-flowing motion far into advanced years have enjoyed sports all their lives and still do calisthenics daily.

If you have been less than lively for a number of years, don't jolt yourself into strenuous athletics immediately. Start off with brisk walks, dancing, bowling, or other accessible sports and gradually advance to more vigorous activities. Resume calisthenics gradually—a few minutes the first day, slowly working up to fifteen or twenty minutes a day. Once begun, be sure you are conscientious about following your exercise program. The reward will be a well-toned, youthfully graceful and lithe figure.

Good posture is important at every age. It's *mandatory* for a mature woman. A youngster should be reprimanded for slumping. A woman can only be reminded of the figure faults it leads to: "dowager's hump" (that unattractive thickening at the nape of the neck), a lumpy middle, round shoulders, jutting head. All these make a body look older than it actually is. Unfortunately, some bodies are actually misshapen by years of bad posture. If you find yourself in this sad shape, don't give up. First, starting at once, practice perfect posture during every waking moment to avoid compounding the faults. Second, do some posture exercises daily to help strengthen the controlling muscles and bring some measure of improvement. Try the good posture habit. See if your figure doesn't look better *instantly* and if you don't feel less tired by the end of the day. Also—and it's a delightful "plus"—your magnificent carriage will give you a "presence" that is apt and attractive for a real woman.

FASHION

Never dress for your age; dress for your type. It's an old maxim and it still goes. Today, women of "a certain age" are often slim and lively enough to wear fashions designed for ingenues—and *do*. There are always qualifications, of course, and a woman is expected to use sound judgment in choosing her fashion. If you can pick up a size seven or nine in the junior department, great. But don't pick up fads that are meant strictly for teenagers. The incongruity of "kiddish" fashion on a mature (albeit well-proportioned) body has an effect of instant aging.

Exposing too much epidermis (except possibly at the beach, pool, or tennis court) should be avoided by most women over fifty, or sometimes before that. It's hard to compete with younger women in the skin game. Skip sleeveless dresses, off the shoulder modes, deep décolletage bare midriffs, halter tops, and thigh-high slits, unless the flesh they reveal is firm, smooth, and even in color. Otherwise, in your fashion, look for what's there—not what's missing. A cocktail or evening dress with sheer flowing sleeves and a high jewel neckline can add far more to your charm than one that puts too much flesh in the open. For daytime, too, long sleeves can combine high fashion with high practicality—especially since elbows and upper arms are tattletales about years. When legs are marked by varicose veins or broken surface veins, wear opaque or textured hose or, when appropriate, pants.

A woman should plan her wardrobe systematically, concentrating on good basics. She must be discerning in her choice, rather than impulsive. A little novelty is fun, but be sure it's right for *you*. Avoid picking up "odds and ends." A woman can't carry off the mistakes of irresistible bargains as easily as a young girl might.

There's a know-how to wearing jewelry—whether it's precious or of the costume variety. Your jewelry is an important fashion accessory and bespeaks your personality, too. Some women can wear an abundance of dramatic jewelry; others prefer the accent of a single classic piece. What and how much you wear depends on your type, your costume, the occasion. Do coordinate your jewelry to your clothes with great care. Costume jewelry is smart, current, and since it doesn't cost a king's ransom, it's simple to buy a new pin, necklace, or earrings to add the right touch to a contemporary outfit.

Watch your color schemes! This becomes more and more important with every passing year. Black and some dark neutrals look too somber on mature women. If you wear them at all, be sure to add a bright or light scarf at your throat, and wear a slightly rosier lipstick, perhaps an extra touch of blush on the cheeks. Some shades of beige and warm browns are attractive basic shades—navy, with light or bright color close to the face is excellent. If your hair is gray, or any pale tone, you will find that pastels, light blues, mauve, corals, are flattering fashion colors.

"At my age, I deserve a little comfort." Some women say it jokingly, but when it comes to apparel, comfort should be considered one of the essentials. There's no need to suffer with ill-fitting clothes. Today's fashions combine chic with great ease. You can't show perfect poise when you must tug or pull at your clothes; your fashion should help, not hinder in this respect.

Select your undergarments with as much care as your most important fashion. The fit and the line they create can make or break everything you wear over them.

Cultivate an eye for the contemporary by reading fashion reports in papers and magazines and by watching others with an analytical eye. If you can't trust your own fashion instinct, find a "model" to follow. It may be an actress, a society figure, the wife of a diplomat, someone who is often pictured in the press or on TV and is not too different from you in personality type and build. You might be guided by watching her skirt lengths and the basic lines she favors. I know several women who have followed this policy and made tremendous strides in their own fashion as a result.

Pay attention to the "little things." Outmoded eye-glass frames can date you in a minute. Wearing shoes that are out of style ("but I wore them only twice and they were expensive. . . .") is a bad mistake. The wrong hat—horrors! Some things in your wardrobe can be carried over from year to year; others are expendable and must go, even if it's a wrench.

Have you noticed the gleam that comes in a young

girl's eye when she passes a dress shop window or leafs through a current magazine? Enjoyment of clothes is a youthful quality. Try to recapture this feeling of excitement in fashion—temper it with your own mature judgment—and you can be sure whatever you wear will add to your lovely appearance.

IS IT YOUR AGE— OR YOUR ATTITUDE?

"It's all in the mind." Is it? Well, not *all,* but a great deal does start with one's mental attitude. What you're thinking works its way to the surface and is revealed to the eyes and ears of the world in gestures, sounds, facial expressions. It's not surprising then that eventually your frame of mind becomes your personality. "What does that have to do with the way I look?" you might ask. A lot, really. Do you realize that your personality is more *visible* as you grow older? A frown, a drooping mouth, sloping shoulders, a slow gait may be fleeting visitors in youth, but if you harbor them long enough they become permanent residents. As much as your conversation, they label you a negative thinker. A pleasant expression, a ready smile, a straight back, and purposeful walk all identify the person in the mainstream of life. If you want to keep youth in your years, you *must* keep optimism and interest in your mental attitude.

Not long ago, we had a farewell party at our New York office for a charming lady who had decided to retire. She had handled an important administrative job with great ability and apparently had enjoyed doing it. In her own magic formula, efficiency was blended with humor and quiet charm. The fact that she had been with the company almost forty years was not evident from her appearance or manner. When she announced her departure one thing that *was* obvious was the reaction of those who had worked with her. Everyone was loath to see her go. At the end of the party, M. H. gave a short speech. "I thought it was time to retire," she said, ". . . since I am getting married tomorrow." Were we surprised? Not very. M. H. was a jewel likely to be discovered. Besides, she had spent her life opening doors and finding something interesting and exciting behind each one. Those who knew her would have been surprised only if she had stopped.

M. H. is not unique. I know late-blooming success stories by the score, and I'm sure you do, too. Marriage is only one of the happy possibilities. Some women find heightened joy in life after shedding a husband! Some mothers, finding the nest empty, switch to a role that demands less self-sacrifice and allows more self-expression. Any number of women, at "middle age" or well past it, return to school, open a business, start a career, sharpen a talent, or move to another part of the world. Life's adventure need never stop, unless you want it to. It's not enough to mouth the words; you must really believe *it's never too late.* Most time limits in life are of our own making. Some impulses must be stifled because they're impractical or not suited to your life-style. Taking up surfing or running off with your dancing teacher, for example. However, don't use age as an excuse. Every time a woman decides she is "too old" for something she is closing a door on life.

Some people start to slam doors shut when they are still young. Then they lock them! These are the people who act old, look old, grow old. If you want to enjoy your years—if you want to be treasured rather than tolerated—keep an open mind. Resisting change, comparing today with yesterday and finding yesterday invariably better, is indicative of a spirit gone flat. You need not accept *all* latest fads, fashion, philosophies, and music, but at least look and listen. Find out what today is all about; what appeals to young people and why. Then, if you *still* don't go along with the new scene, don't sermonize. Maybe some other inhabitants of this planet don't approve of *your* fads, fashions, philosophies, and music. There's room for variety in our world, and it's still the spice of life.

When you open doors and open your mind, you keep freshness and flexibility in your personality. One of the freshest, most flexible women I know has a policy of making what she calls "an important addition" to her life annually. One year (when she was in her sixties!) it was ice skating. Another year it was volunteer work. Last year she learned to play the Spanish guitar. Each new interest brings her a "bonus" of enjoyable new friends. Her zest for living is so contagious, so irresistible, that she is constantly sought after and receives twice as many invitations as she could possibly accept.

People are living longer than ever. And youth is extended further and further into a woman's life. She has within reach every tool and technique for beauty that lasts. She has opportunities galore for meaningful activity. With a beautifully polished appearance and a positive mental attitude, today's woman need never ask, "How old do you think I am?" She feels vital and looks lovely. Isn't that the *perfect* age?

9

Putting It All Together

Assemblage is an art. You can have the perfect ingredients for your chef-d'oeuvre, but without the right mix and timing the results may be shameful. Whether you're putting together a souffle, a dinner party, or a Broadway musical, an eye to detail is important. When it's a question of putting *you* together, it's *de rigueur.*

A schedule is essential, of course. Some women keep theirs in their heads and never skip a beat. Most women, however, do better with a written program—at least until it becomes completely automatic. A basic beauty-grooming routine I had once outlined for college freshmen was requested in duplicate by practically every girl; many mothers wanted copies for their own use and, in instances where they hadn't *asked* for it, their daughters felt the older generation *needed* it.

Here it is then, a checklist suitable for all ages and adaptable to specific needs. A daily check column may seem too great a regimentation—yet it was included at the suggestion of a mature woman who rewarded herself at the end of the week when her score was perfect. When it wasn't, she tried harder.

Whether you check, just glance, or keep all the elements in your mind, do remember that it is *consistency* in beauty grooming that will lead to the well-polished, attractive look you're after.

Morning	SUN.	MON.	TUES.	WED.	THURS.	FRI.	SAT.
Exercise							
Shower							
Deodorant							
Dusting powder/cologne							
Brush teeth							
Mouthwash							
Morning skin care							
Don fresh lingerie							
Apply makeup							
Brush and comb hair							
Complete dressing							
Bedtime							
Do personal laundry: lingerie, gloves							
Select outfit for next day lay out lingerie, accessories							
Check handbag contents							
Brush hair (set if necessary)							
Evening skin care							
Brush teeth							
Hand lotion							

Once a Week (set a definite night for this!)

Shampoo hair, condition
Manicure
Pedicure
Facial mask
Eyebrows—pluck out stragglers
Remove superfluous hair
Luxurious tub bath

YOUR FASHION

Your eye for detail must gaze in many directions. When you're putting yourself together for total attractiveness, take a careful look at your wardrobe. Fads are fleeting, but certain principles of line, style, and color are constant. The eye can be led, and sometimes it can be fooled. Horizontal stripes make any surface look wider. If the surface happens to be your body, don't wear them unless you're slim. Vertical stripes will make you look taller. Dark tones tend to recede an area; light tones bring it forward. If you're top-heavy, with an overlarge bust and slim hips, a dark blouse or jacket with a paler skirt or pants will give more balanced proportions to the beholder's eye. If your hips are too well padded and your bust under-endowed, reverse the order—light color on top, darker below. Anything that cuts across your body breaks the line and stops the eye. A wide belt makes a tall girl appear less so; it's not recommended for a shortie. Your skirt length breaks the line too; within the trend of fashion's dictates, modify your hemline an inch or two to achieve the proportions best for you.

There's no point in being in the height of fashion if it's pointing up a flaw. This is obvious when some rather fat knees are displayed by too short skirt lengths. Be alert to new looks, but temper your choices with awareness of the basic lines, styles, and mood of fashion best suited to your shape and type.

There are trends in fashion that relate to needs and attractiveness, and thus make sense: Pants, for example. They've become a way of life for many women and, in one form or another, belong in practically every wardrobe. With a range of styles, lengths, widths, and looks, there are pants for every figure and every age. Just be sure to suit your choice to your shape. Take a long look, in a triple mirror, at your rear and side view before you buy. If you are the type to indulge in passing fancies, be sure to know when to let them pass.

The woman who draws "best dressed" raves in her own circle isn't necessarily the one who spends the most money. On the contrary, often the one who must accept the enforced restraint of a budget walks off with the fashion honors. She *must* be more organized in her planning. She maps out her wardrobe in great detail, shops with care, substitutes good sense for impulse.

It's important to be a discerning shopper. It's equally important to be a discerning "putter-together." The essence of fashion is interplay. Assembling an outfit with properly balanced accessories, with color harmony, with the right degree of accent, and the most enhancing touch of makeup, makes all the difference between being merely clothed and being à la mode.

Review your wardrobe at the start of each season, culling the good from the gone. Many basics have classic qualities and with the addition of a fresh scarf, belt, or jewelry accent might take a new lease on life. On the other hand, some "hits" of the moment have short runs; when any item of apparel is obviously dated, donate it to a worthy cause. Keeping things you rarely wear, or wear with discomfort, merely clutters your closet and does nothing for your fashion look or morale.

Just as you set aside time for your beauty schedule, be sure to plan a specific time for wardrobe maintenance. Sort out things to go to the cleaner, the shoemaker, the laundry. Use cleaning fluid to remove minor spots, to whisk around the inside of necklines on dresses, the inner bands of your hats. Shine your shoes and polish your leather bags. Check your future plans and appointments and make a note, mental or otherwise, of what you will wear.

Don't forget the *inside* of your handbag; it's as much a part of your fashion as the outside. Many a good impression has changed to bad when an otherwise well-groomed woman has opened her bag and displayed utter chaos within. Or when a woman has pulled out a shabby wallet or beaten-up lipstick case. Your purse accessories should be as attractive as the rest of your fashion, and the inside of your bag should be well arranged, with all of the necessities and none of the superfluities. When you carry a large bag, be sure it holds an "organizer" with handy sleeves into which you can fit cosmetics, keys, notebook, money, etc.

Do you ever finish dressing and realize the bra you put on is all wrong under the knit you're wearing? Or get to the street and find that your slip is riding up under that particular dress which needs the taffeta one? Or decide too late that your hose are the wrong color, or you should have worn the *other* scarf? Few well-dressed women leave it to chance. The busiest ones save time and stress by charting each complete outfit—from the invisible lingerie to the most visible accessories.

CULTIVATING YOUR TOTAL LOOK

Only when you know the exact current condition of your skin, your hair, your figure, can you give each the specific care that will bring it to its best, keep it at its best. We've talked earlier about analyzing these separate parts. Now what about the whole—the complete, coordinated *you?*

Putting oneself together perfectly so that the impression projected is not merely good but *great*, requires careful attention and even artistry. Everything you are— your personality as well as your physical shape—must blend with everything you put on—your makeup, clothes, accessories, hair style—to form a homogeneous and magnificent whole.

Here's an example of a practical chart to be filled in at the beginning of each new season and tacked up inside your closet. A quick glance saves pondering and avoids mistakes in assemblage.

FASHION ORGANIZER

Basic Outfit (Dress, Suit or Pants)	Lingerie	Hose	Blouse Scarf Belt	Jewelry	Shoes	Handbag	Hat	Gloves	Coat	Makeup	Fragrance

The first step is to acknowledge your strengths and weaknesses of appearance. Then you must decide what to accent and what to play down—and how to do it. I see many girls who have even features, well-proportioned figures, all the attributes for good looks—but they fail to register. Everything is "nice" but nothing stands out. They need to dramatize their looks. Others lose their beauty character because they emphasize *everything:* hair is elaborately styled, all makeup too defined, clothes too fussy or overbright, accessories and jewelry too dominant. Every picture has a focal point—so does every attractive woman. Find yours and make it the star of your appearance; let your other features play the obbligato.

A woman who manages a small boutique in Paris could be rather undistinguished looking—if it weren't for her bright blue eyes. She plays them up for all they're worth! Her eye makeup is a subtle work of art, and every time I have seen her she has been wearing blue, or a soft shade of gray with a pretty blue scarf at the throat. Very cleverly, she wears only one piece of jewelry—a sapphire ring. She knows how to make the most of an asset!

Many smart women "play to type." This is a favorite device of actresses and models who must make a strong impression or want to be remembered in a specific way. As a general rule, I believe that "type" evolves naturally. One wears the clothes, the hairstyle, the makeup that suit one's looks, preferences, activities—and the image is a valid reflection of the person. Today's woman is so versatile that she doesn't fit easily into categories; in fact, one woman may change her "type" several times a day, depending on the hour, the occasion, the companion.

However, any woman who is dissatisfied with her present look and who is seeking a total look that is more expressive of her personality should study herself not only from head to toe but from the inside out to determine whether she is projecting her character and whether she is emphasizing her physical attributes to best advantage. Having your own hallmark—something that you're "famous" for—is a great contributor to an individual look, provided it is entirely right for you. A delightful young Englishwoman is known among her friends as "the suit girl." She wears practically nothing *but* suits. Depending upon the time and place, she may be seen in tweedy suits, tailored suits, cocktail suits, well coordinated jackets and skirts, or a velvet blazer with floor-length skirt. She told me that she felt "tall, plain, and lonely" when she moved to London from a small village in Devon. "Frankly, I started wearing separates because they gave me more fashion versatility on a limited budget," she explained. "But then I realized that skirts and tops broke my long thin line and made me look better proportioned. So that I wouldn't look oversevere, I let my hair grow shoulder length to minimize my long neck, then I lightened it for fun. When I was invited to my first big evening party in London, I tried on dress after dress. My shoulders looked all bones, I was flat as a pancake, and I appeared seven feet tall! In desperation I bought a long black skirt and wore a white linen jacket with it. I was the most covered-up female at the party—but I felt marvelously comfortable. I felt like *me.* And I got so much attention that night—including my sobriquet—that I decided to adopt suits for good!" Delightfully, no one dreams she wears suits to camouflage her lankiness. They "suit" her personality, that's all!

USING COLOR POWER

Color influences moods and motivation; it calms or excites; it appeals or repels. Color has power! Have you put that power to work for you? A personal color scheme that blends skintone, hair, makeup, fashion, in delightful harmony contributes a great deal to the unity of your total look and certainly to your total attractiveness!

With the right makeup, you can wear practically *any* color. But why should you? In the vast spectrum there are a number of hues that complement your natural coloring—your skin, your hair, your eyes. These are the colors that "do things" for you—that accent the lovely lights in your hair, reflect a radiance in your complexion, emphasize the sparkling color of your eyes. Then there are the colors that do all the wrong things—make your skin appear sallow or overflorid, dull your good looks and create discord.

Every woman should know, without question, the friendly shades that pay homage to her beauty, and should recognize enemies. The list of "flatterers" should include neutrals, basic colors, pastels, and accents, and the woman who uses color advantageously will choose only from her flattering group. How does one determine one's best colors? Because of the great diversity of personal coloring and fashion's endless color mutations, a practiced eye is generally the best guide. Before you try a dress on, hold it against you—close to your face—and see what it does to your skin, eyes, hair. If it complements them all, well and good. If it dulls or overpowers, the color is not for you, nor is the dress, regardless of its fit and lines.

I hate hard and fast rules—especially in relation to color, which should be chosen with delight rather than by decree. However, there are a few fundamentals one must keep in mind.

Brilliant colors can overpower unless your *own* coloring is dramatic. Don't wear them if you're fair-skinned, blond, or gray. They're too apt to wash *you* out.

Tones with a yellowish or muddy hue—chartreuse, mustard, maroon—are not for the sallow-skinned. Try clear blue, green, rose-pink and limit black and gray to accessories.

Bright pinks, fuchsia, electric blue reflect too much radiance in an overflorid skin. Muted tones, rosewood, pastels, greens help "cool" it.

Cold colors—black, gray, blue, and lavender—emphasize "tired," dull skin and any darkness under the eyes. Break their frigid grasp with a light or bright-toned scarf.

Color belongs in your fashion and your fashion is part of your beauty. Keeping all in harmony takes careful study, time discipline. That well-dressed woman who was never known to make a shopping mistake, whose every choice is a triumph, maps out her wardrobe strategy as carefully as a general on the offensive. She follows fashion magazines and newspapers; she studies window displays; she clips pictures of possibilities for future purchase; she juggles what she owns with what she needs; she leaves little to chance. And she doesn't waste money. Following fashion rules instead of impulse is the best deterrent to filling your closet with little bargains you bought on the spur of the moment but which drain your budget and add nothing to your good looks.

YOUR VOICE AND YOU

It might be quite invisible, but your voice is such an important part of *you* and of the total impression you create. A soft, gentle, low voice, as Shakespeare pointed out, is quite an asset.

A serious problem or deeply imbedded habit of bad speech will need the professional help of a speech therapist or voice teacher. Most women, however, don't have serious problems. I have noticed that there are two principal faults which, fortunately, can be corrected with just a little effort.

First is shrillness. Women have a higher pitch than men. When a man raises his voice he booms; when a woman raises hers she shrieks. The answer, of course, is *don't shout*. A friend of mine who lives in the country has a bell which she rings to summon her children—for meals, for phone calls, for any reason. Until she turned to the bell, she used to bellow—and, as with many mothers, this became a habit. Not only would she bellow to call the children indoors, she would bellow from one room to the other, she would bellow up and down the stairs, and finally one day when she found herself bellowing at the table the children, all at the same time, put their fingers in their ears. That was when she was shocked into adopting the bell system and made a vow not to raise her voice to a bellow ever again.

Unless you're warning someone from the path of an enraged bull, shouting serves no purpose. A firm, strong voice conveys even the most urgent message and can carry over a considerable distance when necessary. Next time you feel impelled to yell, think of the actresses whose tender words on stage carry to the last row of the balcony. If you're on a noisy train, in a restaurant or nightclub where music or hubbub drown out your words, don't try to converse with shrieks. Give up until the noise is over.

The second fault is sloppiness. One picks up slang expressions, runs words together, or fails to value the sound of her own voice. "Wanna," "gonna," "didja," "uh-huh" are sprinkled through the vocabulary and excess verbiage such as "you know" or "you see?" is tacked on the end of each sentence. The tone falls flat—and so does the conversation.

Listen to your own voice now and then. Watch the pitch, the enunciation, the choice of words. Don't assume an accent that isn't your own, of course, but do improve what you've got. Actresses read aloud to themselves as an exercise in projection and improving vocal quality. Why don't you try it occasionally? It's a marvelous way to reread the classics, your favorite poetry, or to absorb the editorial page in the evening paper.

What you say is also part of your total impression, and —whatever it is—it sounds more interesting when your voice is pleasant. The art of conversation, well-cultivated in times past, is free form today. Talk that springs from interest, involvement, and zest for living doesn't need structure or stylized form. Remember always, though, that some of the women who win praise as great conversationalists are the best listeners. There's an art to listening—not merely hearing sounds but comprehending the message and being sincerely interested. There's always the temptation to "top" someone else's story, to be impatient to express your own opinion or views. Every now and then, just for a change, resist the temptation. Give the other person a chance to expound. Ask a few questions. Comment on *his* conversation. And *then,* if you wish, launch into your own. Above all, don't talk just for the sake of talking. Speech, as silvery as it may be, becomes dull idle chatter if what you're expressing is of no interest to your listener.

The way you sound, the way you look, the way you move—even the haunting fragrance you wear—every detail is part of the composite picture that becomes YOU. Putting everything together perfectly can be a great adventure. There's anticipation in drawing up your own beauty and fashion plan. There's enlightenment in following it. And, of course, there is great reward in achieving your goal. The total woman who evolves is the you who was meant to be—not a reasonable facsimile of a movie star or a carbon copy of your best friend; not someone whose own identity is smothered under an assumed character—but YOU, looking your best, projecting your own one-in-the-world personality. And what could be more worth the effort than *that?*

10

A Day of Beauty

WHAT IT'S LIKE AT A LUXURIOUS SALON AND HOW TO PLAN YOUR OWN AT HOME

Ellen, a bright young attorney, and I had met at several functions. She was a study in perrpetual motion—professional busy, involved in community projects, member of several philanthropic and alumni committees, and always eager for special projects. It seemed Ellen found time for everything—except herself.

On one occasion, Ellen and I shared the platform at a fund-raising luncheon. As we were leaving, she made an amusing comment about her hair (it really didn't do her justice) and added, "I know I should spend a day at your salon, but to me that's like the grapes were to Tantalus—always out of reach." I started to ask why, but Ellen was already nervously checking the time and murmuring about "unnecessary luxury" and "priorities."

Not long after, I had a phone call from a long-time acquaintance, who was a partner in the same law firm as Ellen. He told me she had just won a complex case out of town. As a welcome-back, the partners had decided to give her a Day of Beauty at the Helena Rubinstein Salon.

Ellen—always diligent—never ignored an appointment! Her day at our salon unfolded as follows.

9:30   First, a diet and exercise expert discussed with

Ellen the exercises she should do daily to firm certain areas and improve her general fitness. Her measurements, and the ones she should aim for, were written on a chart she would take with her—along with a chart of diet suggestions —on leaving.

10:00   Ellen changed into a leotard and tights. As soon as she entered the attractive gym, she was told by the exercise expert to "start stretching." Holding her arms straight up, she stretched higher and higher. "Now stretch to the sides—further—further!" After showing Ellen how to warm up her muscles for exercise, the instructor demonstrated the exercises that were recommended specifically for her needs. Next she tossed a beach ball to Ellen and showed her a fun exercise for a great overall "tune-up."

Standing back to back with the instructor, legs apart, Ellen bent forward from the waist and passed the ball through her legs to the teacher, who brought the ball forward and up with straight arms, stretching high overhead. Ellen took the ball from overhead and brought it down again, repeating the circle a number of times.

The half hour passed quickly. Ellen could feel that her arms, waist, abdomen muscles had benefited—and decided that exercise could be great fun, too.

10:30   Next, Ellen was shown into a private salon bathroom where a deep tub was filled with warm water. She caught the fragrance of an herbal bath oil. As she let her body down into the tub, she felt the caressing water smooth her skin. A fresh cake of perfumed soap was at hand. On a chair, a thick-piled towel, a terry robe, and slippers awaited her emergence from the bath. She had been told to relax, and she did! After drying her body and donning the robe, she was ready for her body massage.

11:00 In the massage room, Ellen felt every last bit of tension fade away under the firm, expert hands of the masseuse. Special attention was given to the back of Ellen's neck, the area between the shoulder blades, and the spine area—places where Ellen told the masseuse she would feel "knotted up in nervousness" on a demanding business day. Before the massage was finished, Ellen confided that she hadn't felt so "blissful" in ages. Surprising herself, Ellen became sleepy, so we allowed her to take a fifteen-minute nap after the massage. (And we had been afraid she might become restless!)

12:00 Ellen was given a salon robe, coral, trimmed with gold, to wear for the rest of her Day of Beauty. She said that the soft color gave her a lift but that mostly she appreciated the unfettered comfort she felt in it and in her little paper slippers.

12:15 Lunch is served in a small private dining room, bright with sunshine. There are fresh flowers on Ellen's luncheon tray. The food is calorie-counted, attractively arranged on fine china, and delicious.

12:45 A session with the salon fashion consultant was optional, but Ellen decided to include a consultation after lunch. She told the consultant that she was spending quite a lot for clothes but didn't feel she had achieved a fashion "look." The consultant pointed out the lines and shapes that would make Ellen look taller and thinner (just what she wanted) and recommended the colors that would add interest and drama. She explained how Ellen could pull her wardrobe together in terms of outfits; how to mix pieces for variety and convenience during business travels; and how to choose and use accessories. She promised to draw up Ellen's own fashion plan and give it to her before she left the salon.

1:00   Next came the Face Treatment. Ellen stretched out on an adjustable reclining chair. The Face Treatment operator, expert in every area of skin care, examined Ellen's skin under a magnifying glass. She found it to be in good condition, but with a scattering of clogged pores and blackheads. The type of face treatment given depends on the individual's need. Ellen was given a Deep Pore Treatment to clear the pores of impurities and refine the skin; this was followed by a rich lubricating treatment for the dry skin areas. The final touch—a refreshing facial mask. Ellen was given instructions on caring for her skin at home and emphatic advice: "For your skin—no sun. And stop frowning; you'll make lines." "I'm not frowning *now,*" Ellen told the operator. "In fact, I'm floating on a cloud!"

2:00   Ellen was escorted to the Hair Salon, where an expert stylist studied her hair and facial structure, asked her about her activities, her own handling of her hair, and made a suggestion that delighted Ellen. After his assistant had shampooed and conditioned Ellen's hair, the stylist clipped and shaped to create an exciting new coiffure. As well as being wonderfully attractive, it was a style that Ellen could easily handle herself, at home or while traveling.

3:00   A manicurist and a pedicurist arrived just before the hair-drying process began. Now Ellen had the delicious feeling of being waited on "hand and foot—and head, too!" Before its final combing, Ellen's hair was drawn off her face and protected with a headband.

4:00   She's ready for makeup! The makeup artist studied Ellen's personal coloring and the structure and shape of her face. He asked her what fashion colors she generally wore. Then he told her in advance the makeup look he planned to create. In Ellen's case, the artist felt that a pale blue on the lid, with deep plum shadow blended subtly on the edge of the bone, would "bring out" her deep-set eyes. He explained how he would contour her cheekbones with a tawny blush and give her lips a fuller look with two shades of lipstick. Ellen wanted to close her eyes while he worked his magic, but the artist urged her to watch every step. "So that you can duplicate them when you apply your own makeup," he told her.

4:30   Makeup finished, headband removed, Ellen's hair was given its final combing. She can't believe her reflection in the mirror! Even more, she can't believe how relaxed, how happy she feels. "I've just discovered a new priority," she told me when I stopped by to see her before she left. "It's *me!*"

4:45   But wait, Ellen! There's one more thing before you go. A salon assistant presented a neat pink folder—Ellen's "souvenir" of the day, and her guide to many more beautiful days. In the folder: diet charts, exercise charts, calorie-counted suggested menus, daily skin care advice, a how-to makeup guide—even a fashion plan—all personally planned for Ellen. A wonderful way to end a Day of Beauty and start the care that means a beautiful lifetime.

YOUR OWN DAY OF BEAUTY

Everyone can't have a Day of Beauty at a luxurious salon, but the busier a woman is, the more she needs to set aside time for herself—for taking care of her face and body, and putting aside the stress and worries of every day. It's wonderful therapy, and it's in every woman's reach.

If you don't live alone, choose a day when no one else will be home. Send your spouse or roommate off on a fishing trip; give the kids a wonderful day out with their favorite aunt! Only complete and uninterrupted privacy will give you the feeling of total relaxation that's part of the plan.

In advance, check to be sure you have everything you need: beauty supplies, the right food, a fresh robe and leotards. Put everything in easy reach. Rummaging for a missing element can spoil the mood. Bring in fresh flowers the day before. *Your* Day of Beauty is going to be beautiful!

HERE'S YOUR PLAN:

Sleep a little later if you like this morning and eat a very light breakfast. Resolve today to refresh your body, inside as well as out, by eating lightly, drinking only juices and mineral water. Avoid cigarettes, coffee, tea, snacks, and so forth throughout the day.

9:30 Cleanse and freshen your face. Use a little lip gloss.

9:45 Appraise your figure. Weigh yourself and check your dimensions with a tape measure. Jot down the numbers on your record card. Keep this to mark the progress you make from month to month.

10:00 Don your leotards, put on your favorite music, and enjoy half an hour of the exercises best for you.

10:30 Take a beauty bath! Make it long and luxurious. Use a bath oil if your skin is dry, bubble bath if it isn't. While you're lolling in the tub, sip mineral water with a twist of lemon from a champagne or wine glass. After your bath, while your skin is still slightly damp, smooth on a fragrant body lotion. Massage it well into feet, elbows, other dry spots. As soon as your skin has absorbed the lotion, put on a pretty robe.

11:00 Give yourself the perfect pedicure. Be sure the final touch is nail enamel in a bewitching shade. While your nails are drying, stretch comfortably on a chaise longue (or your couch) and lazily look through the latest fashion magazines.

11:30 With pad and pencil, note ways to update your wardrobe. Just think and plan—no rearranging of closets today!

12:00 Lunch time. With fresh flowers on the table and an attractively arranged salad on your plate, eat at a leisurely pace. After lunch, read something delightful for half an hour.

1:00 Treat your face. Tie up your hair and follow the skin care plan recommended in this book for your skin type. Cleanse, freshen, pat eye cream around your eyes. If your skin is dry, smooth a rich emollient over face and throat. Leave it on ten to fifteen minutes; then remove any residue by wiping upward and outward with cotton pad saturated with freshener. Next: a facial mask. While it's on your face, stretch out with your feet raised on a pillow. Cover your eyes with cotton pads saturated with herbal lotion or freshener. Now, for 20 to 30 minutes, pretend you're floating on a cloud. After you remove the mask, sip another glass of mineral water.

2:00 Massage your scalp, brush your hair, shampoo

and condition. Do a thorough job—today you're special! Give extra time to styling, so that it looks professionally done.

3:00 Attend to your hands. Give them a good massage with rich cream. Then soak your fingernails in warm olive oil for fifteen minutes. Wipe off excess oil and cream, and follow the steps for a perfect manicure (see the "hands" section in this book). While your nail enamel is drying, listen to the music you love. Enjoy a glass of vegetable or fruit juice.

4:00 Put on your most enchanting makeup. Try new colors, new effects, perhaps. Follow all the special techniques to enhance your individual good looks. Now, lavish on the cologne you've been saving for special occasions or touch perfume to your pulse spots.

4:30 Dress for the evening, whatever you've planned. And enjoy yourself—looking as though you had just returned from a refreshing holiday—or spent the day at a luxurious salon!

11

"Dear Miss Rubinstein"

"Dear Miss Rubinstein, I would like to know . . ."
How many times have I read those words! Over the years, letters have poured in from all over the world, asking advice or comments, and countless questions have been asked vis-à-vis. I love questions and person-to-person contact. I value them, too, as they are indicative of trends and composite interest.

As Kipling pointed out, we are all "sisters under the skin." This is never more apparent than in the daily mail, when a problem expressed in a letter from a girl in Singapore may be repeated in a communication received the same morning from a woman in Muskogee, Oklahoma. Some subjects on which I receive frequent inquiries are of interest to many, many women, and so I have dug into my "grab bag" of letters and questions and selected a few to share with you.

"Dear Miss Rubinstein:
My new job involves a lot of travel—even overseas, where the local representatives of my company generally meet me at the airport on my arrival. Naturally, I want to look my best. So far, I'm afraid it has been the

contrary. Any tips on how to arrive looking good after an overnight flight?"

I know exactly how you feel. A long plane trip, particularly one that crosses time zones and throws off one's internal clock, can leave the traveler feeling worn—and showing it. With a little planning, however, you can step off the plane as attractive and well-groomed as when you embarked.

Try to organize all your activities, your packing, your social schedule, so that the last day before departure is free from rush and tension. Insist on getting a good sleep the night before. On the day of departure, apply your makeup with a light touch. Heavy makeup may become caked and looks "tired" very quickly. Choose a simple hair style that won't be too badly disturbed by being pressed against the headrest for some hours.

Of course your travel outfit will be smart but wrinkle-proof. I find that belts or waistbands dig in after several hours, so I choose a semifitted or A-line dress rather than separates of any kind. A jacket dress is good at most seasons. Remove the jacket as soon as you get on the plane and let it hang until you're ready to disembark. Carry an extra pair of gloves and a gay scarf in your flight bag for use on arrival.

Your flight bag should hold small sizes of a lotion cleanser, skin freshener, moisturizer, tissues, cotton pads, premoistened paper towelettes, cologne spray, and a small mirror (perhaps a double-faced kind, with one side magnifying). Be sure to include all essential makeup items either in your flight bag or handbag. You might add a pair of folding slippers to change to after takeoff. In flight you can let your flight bag double as a footstool; elevating the feet helps avoid possible swelling. Since sitting in one position for many hours is bad for the circulation, stand up now and then and stretch. After you finish your overnight snooze, try the following body stretches, which you can do quite inconspicuously right in your seat: Slip off your shoes and curl your toes under, then stretch them out. Raise feet a few inches off the floor and press the heels down as far as possible. Stretch one leg way out, feeling tension from toes to thighs; then relax that leg and stretch the other. Pull in your stomach, pressing your back against the seat. Stretch your spine from base to top, ending with a good neck stretch, pulling your head up as high as you can. Clasp your hands in your lap and stretch both arms toward the knees. All these stretches will help dispel any stiff feeling.

Before landing, cleanse and freshen your face. If possible, use your lotion cleanser; otherwise, quick-cleanse with skin freshener on a cotton pad. Don't disturb your eye makeup. Cleanse around it. Carefully applied shadow, liner, mascara, and brow makeup should survive the trip beautifully. Apply moisturizer and foundation (use a non-spillable foundation stick). Add translucent face powder (pressed compact form) and a touch of blush on your cheekbones. Be sure all old lipstick is removed and apply fresh color to your lips. Wipe off your hands with the pre-moistened towelettes. Spray cologne on your wrists, the back of your neck, your arms (if bare), the palms of your hands.

Be sure to include a breath freshener in your flight bag or handbag. A small spray type is convenient when the "fasten seat belts" sign precludes a trip to the washroom.

Now—walk off the plane, looking polished and poised and ready to meet your welcoming committee with confidence.

"Dear Miss Rubinstein:
Do you think women should be completely deprived of makeup when going to bed—especially someone like me who looks completely washed out without it? This didn't bother me until recently, but as the man I am going to marry likes to see me at my best . . ."

There's no need to give your man too great a shock.

You *can* look pretty at bedtime, but not with a lot of makeup. Your face needs to get undressed at night, just as your body does, and it can be very attractive in its "for his eyes only" role.

You mustn't neglect your evening skin-care ritual, but you need not go to bed with a greased-up face. At nighttime, cleanse your face thoroughly and follow with skin freshener. Apply your lubricating cream before the bath or before you take care of a few nighttime grooming details in the bathroom, and it will practically disappear into your skin in a matter of minutes. Some of the richest, most emollient creams are quickly absorbed. Blot the surface if there is any shiny residue.

If your eyes need accent, use a light touch of liner: blue, gray, or light brown are quiet bedtime shades. Brush your brows and use eyebrow pencil very lightly if they need definition or filling in. Use a transparent lip gloss, with just a hint of color, on your lips. If you are very pale and feel you must have a vague blush, use a light glow of transparent color on your cheekbones. Spray on a fragrant cologne—and wear something fetchingly female. You're ready for bed—and you're beautiful!

Once you take up residence with a man, make a vow to create beautiful illusions—not shatter them. Every man knows that beauty needs a few props, but he would rather this be part of the "feminine mystique"—not cold facts thrown in his face. Few things are more chilling to romance than a head full of rollers. Unconfined, free-flowing hair looks pretty on a pillow. If at all possible, adopt a hairstyle that doesn't require nightly pinups. If you *must* put your hair up at night, cover the evidence with a pretty chiffon scarf or a turban of tulle. Or you can depend on a set of fast-acting heat-activated rollers. Make it a rule to apply and remove makeup away from your man's gaze. Don't leave your false eyelashes sitting on the dressing table like a couple of tarantulas on the loose. Your at-home wardrobe should be comfortable, but be sure it's attractive, too.

Brushing the teeth, gargling, tweezing the eyebrows—the many things that make you a lovely woman—are not necessarily lovely to behold. The happiest relationships give each partner freedom to attend to intimate grooming chores in complete privacy. This needn't mean taking over the bathroom for long hours, but it might mean rearranging your schedule a little. Living with a man requires some adjustment, it's true—but most women agree it's well worth the challenge!

"Dear Miss Rubinstein:
Do you ever recommend plastic surgery? It used to be a hush-hush subject, but now it's discussed so openly. What do you think?"

I certainly do recommend plastic surgery but only when I consider it absolutely necessary for the person's appearance and morale. I don't believe any surgery (including plastic) should be entered into without very good reason. Plastic surgery is expensive, there is an aftermath of discomfort, if not pain, for a period that may range from days to weeks, and there is a certain finality. If the results aren't quite what you had hoped for, there is little you can do about it. By starting correct daily skin care early and avoiding abuse (overexposure to the sun and extremes of weight gain and loss are prime examples), many women can eliminate the need for plastic surgery. Others who have serious structural flaws, or whose facial condition has gone far beyond the help of cosmetic treatment, are well-advised to seek the help of newest surgical methods.

"Dear Miss Rubinstein:
Please tell me about the different kinds of plastic surgery, how long it takes, how long it lasts, and so forth."

Plastic surgery falls into two categories: corrective and restorative.

CORRECTIVE PLASTIC SURGERY—the reshaping of a nose, jawline, ears, chin—is generally done in early adulthood. When a feature seriously detracts from one's appearance, the cost and inconvenience of corrective surgery are far outweighed by the advantages to be gained. It has given a beautiful life to young men and women who otherwise might have existed miserably. Correcting flaws is advantageous; indulging in whims is not. Many a young woman decides she wants a new nose, as casually as if she were making up her mind to have her hair cut. Nose jobs, unlike haircuts, are forever.

Times without number, I have advised *against* plastic surgery when I felt the adjustment of a feature would detract from the character and strength of the face. Sometimes I have a nightmare in which everyone in the world undergoes plastic surgery—one after the other, millions upon millions, rolling along the human assembly line with the same so-called symmetrical features. How grateful I am that we are spared this uniformity! In reality, tiny doll-like features are lovely on tiny, doll-like creatures. They wouldn't suit all of us, however, either to wear or to observe. Some of the most dynamic, most desirable women in the world laugh at symmetry. Their features may be "imperfect" according to well-measured standards. Yet their faces are full of life and interest.

If you're not satisfied with every plane of your face, take another look. If you find more drama than conformity, think of the actresses who turned such dilemma into big box office. Before you move toward corrective surgery, try a new image. You might need a different fashion look. Try "reshaping" your face with makeup. Experiment with hair styles; a change of coiffure might balance your features to better proportion. After these attempts, if you find the feature still offensive, your next step is to find a reputable plastic surgeon. Don't take chances. This could be the big decision of your life. Ask your own doctor or your local medical association to make a recommendation.

RESTORATIVE PLASTIC SURGERY. This technique is the age-dropper that doesn't change the features, but attempts to return the contour to the look it had ten or fifteen years earlier. Generally, it is an after-fifty resort, although it may be called for earlier in some cases. Who needs a face lift? Certainly not every woman. We all grow older but the hand of time is often gentle. The face that has been kept attractively firm and smooth through good health, consistently maintained weight, and attentive skin treatment, can wear its years as compliments. There are some faces, however, that time insults with pouches beneath the eyes, deep furrows from the corners of the nose to the mouth, a slacck contour and flabbiness of the throat. If these signs of time come long before they should, if the man or woman is in the public eye, or works in a highly competitive youth-conscious field, or if his morale and outlook are influenced by his deteriorating appearance, plastic surgery is the logical answer.

Anyone considering this step, I repeat, should realize that a face lift is expensive, time-consuming, and uncomfortable for a time. The cost, length of hospitalization, and recuperative period depend on the extent of the surgery and on the individual's "snap-back" power. Localized attention—just the eye area, for example—may mean an overnight stay in the hospital, a week in hibernation while bruising and swelling subside, back in circulation in about ten days—probably with dark glasses for another week or so. A complete face lift—including face, eyes, throat,—may mean two or three days in the hospital, a couple of weeks of not wanting to look in your mirror, and two to four weeks (depending on your rate of healing) before the debut of your new face. The isolation period does have its advantage. If the lift is a good one, you won't look radically different— just younger and better. If you don't wish to confide, friends will think your "long vacation" did you a world of good.

Does it last a lifetime? Corrective surgery, such as nose remodeling or other structural change, does. However, restorative surgery doesn't. The same forces that caused the sag or lines in the first place are still at work, and a "repair job" may be necessary in time. For some women this may be five years after initial surgery; for others ten. Much depends on your age, the degree of natural firmness and flexibility in your skin, the cosmetic care you give your skin. Skin that is neglected shows signs of age far sooner than well-tended skin and is more apt to need plastic surgery. *After* surgery consistent skin care can help keep the complexion lovely and certainly delay the need for further restorative attention.

> *"Dear Miss Rubinstein:*
> *Can you please help me settle a family dispute? My little sister (14) wants to start using makeup. My mother is against it because she thinks Karen is too young. I don't want her to have to put it on once she's a good distance from the house and take it off before getting home, like I did."*

In most parts of the United States, the average age for using just a little lipstick in public is thirteen. However, some girls don't feel the urge or need for any makeup until several years later; some start experimenting when they are twelve. No one can give a precise age. A great deal depends on the girl, the mores of the community, where and why she would wear makeup, and—of vital importance to teenagers—what "everybody" is doing.

Many parents are overrigid on the subject. Mothers attach historical significance to the fact that they first wore lipstick at sixteen (or fifteen or fourteen) and feel a timeless tradition was thus established. And dismissed from memory are the family protests it provoked! Parents, whether they admit it or not, hate to see their babies grow up. When a girl first shows her face with makeup, her unspoken message is, "Look at me—I'm no longer a child!" Instead of joining her in celebration, parents seem to enter a period of mourning. Keeping a girl away from makeup, once she wants it, is like hiding a razor from your son because you won't admit he's old enough to shave. It doesn't work. A negative parental attitude often drives girls to what I call "rebellious makeup"—defiant, blatant, and not at all pretty.

Girls today have a better sense of makeup than their mothers and grandmothers did; they choose it more intelligently and use it more skillfully. They know that a natural look points up their own beauty and is their best bet. Also, today there are colors and products designed especially for *youth.* A transparent lip gloss with just a trace of color doesn't look "made up," yet it protects lips from chapping and sunburn. A girl with pretty skin prefers to show it, not cover it. If she needs a little color, she will add a glow at the cheekbone only. However, a teenager—regardless of her exact years—whose skin shows excess oiliness and pimples should wear a skin-matching makeup lotion that helps heal while it covers blemishes and improves the appearance of the skin.

Eye makeup is ludicrous on a girl in her early teens. If she is panting for it, give her an appropriate alternative; help her to groom her brows by plucking out "stragglers," show her how to brush her lashes to encourage growth and sweep, let her smooth eye cream across her upper lid for gloss. On girls under seventeen, obvious eye makeup by day is more likely to detract than add appeal. (The exception may be a discreet eyebrow accent if a girl is very fair.) However, by mid-teens a girl who *wants* eye makeup should be taught how to apply shadow, liner, mascara, in subtle colors, for evening parties, holidays, or very special occasions.

It's normal and healthy for a girl to want to look pretty. In many cases, a little makeup imparts a lot of confidence and leads to more attention from boys and, consequently, a happier girl. What she often needs is understanding and a helping hand in selecting the right makeup and using it properly. And a good example doesn't hurt. If you are a mother who wishes to speak with authority on the subject, be sure your *own* makeup is attractive, up-to-date, in good taste for every occasion, and completely right for *you*.

> *"Dear Miss Rubinstein:*
> *The other night I overheard someone telling my steady, 'If she's going to look like her mother later, better forget it.' I was terribly hurt and I'm also worried. I bear a strong resemblance to my mother, at least the way old photographs show her. . . ."*

There's an old European saying that if a man wants to know what his wife will be like in twenty years he should take a good look at her mother. An attractive mother can be a girl's best advertisement; an unattractive one can "unsell" a romance. The mother who fails to impress favorably is often one who has put the material interests of her husband and children before her own. She is the woman who would forgo a new dress, make do with outdated eyeglass frames, skip a needed visit to the hairdresser, and then compensate by having another piece of pie. Self-sacrifice is noble when it is truly necessary; too often, however, it is a handy label that covers carelessness. Mothers should never forget that one of the greatest gifts they can offer their children is pride. Offspring, young and old, want their mothers to be attractive and admired.

The remark you overheard can help you. Since you realize you have a strong resemblance to your mother, and perhaps some inherent traits, analyze the appearance that prompted the remark and start at once to avoid the same faults. Is your mother too heavy because of poorly balanced diet? Is her posture bad? Did she neglect her skin? What's wrong with her makeup, her hair, her fashion? Be extra careful of your own appearance so that your "steady" will be convinced you'll never slip into careless habits.

Very important—don't pass your hurt on to your

mother. It will serve no purpose. Instead, encourage her—gently but kindly—to take care of her skin, to try a new makeup, to take pride in her appearance. For her next birthday, or for no special reason, treat her to a salon appointment for a new hairdo, give her a big bottle of cologne, or the cosmetics she should be using. You can rekindle her desire to be attractive—it's never too late—and give her a new lease on life. And you'll be doing yourself a favor at the same time!

"Dear Miss Rubinstein:
Lately I hear a lot about 'natural cosmetics' that can be made from 'natural ingredients' found in the refrigerator. How do these cosmetics compare with the commercial kind?"

With "natural ingredients" as with anything else, much depends on the ingredient and the individual. One cannot generalize. Some have good effect and are fun to use. Splashing milk on the face, putting rose petals in the tub, using diluted lemon juice as a final rinse after shampooing blonde hair, soaking the nails in warm olive oil are uses of "natural ingredients" that have gone on for years.

However, a number of natural ingredients, in their original form, are messy, smelly, or unpleasant to touch. Some can irritate the skin. Without needed preservatives, the ingredients in home formulas may turn sour, rotten, or rancid, resulting in considerable waste. They rarely travel well as they can't withstand changes of climate, temperature, or altitude. Where do you find the facilities for preparing another batch when your own kitchen is not accessible? To all these problems, add the time and effort involved and then decide if it's worth it. Blending and cooking cosmetic concoctions at home takes us back to great-grandmother's day. The result, at best, cannot compare with the modern cosmetic prepared by expert chemists in scientific laboratories.

Herbs, vegetable extracts, seaweed derivatives, plant

oils, and other natural ingredients are included in our cosmetic formulas. However, they are processed to secure a concentration of the most valuable elements, and then the concentration is balanced with other ingredients to assure ease of application, effective assimilation, and greatest benefit.

A reputable cosmetic company employs dermatologists, pharmacists, biologists, chemists, and specialists in each phase of beauty. It has costly, specially designed equipment in its research laboratories and production centers. It maintains a scrupulous quality-control check. It has every facility for producing the most effective beauty products—and the incentive to do so, for only by thoroughly pleasing its clients can a company retain its business.

> *"Dear Miss Rubinstein:*
> *I'm concerned about the high cost of beauty today. As a working woman on a budget, I need and want to look my best, but I can't afford all the cosmetics recommended."*

Of course the cost of beauty has gone up—everything has. However, it is still one of the best buys around. Be discerning in your selection of skin treatment and makeup products; the greatest extravagance is the purchase of a cosmetic which is ineffective for you because it doesn't serve your specific need. Buy a quality product that is right for you. It will deliver what it promises and give great value with each application. Don't waste. I find that many women use creams and lotions too lavishly. It's not necessary. A little will go a long way.

If you have a budget problem, consider your cosmetics in relation to other outlay. I was amused recently when a woman who is a chain smoker made a similar comment. The amount she spends on cigarettes in one year would more than cover all her cosmetics, makeup, perfume, and bath products! You might find it easy to give up the extra cup of coffee and pastry at break time, to walk instead of taking the bus for short hops, to skip desserts at lunch and put the money in your cosmetic piggy bank. Not only will the savings pay for all your cosmetics—your figure will benefit, too!

"Dear Miss Rubinstein:
I have to start wearing glasses. Can you give me some tips on selecting frames? Also, what about my eye makeup once I wear glasses?"

Today's glasses are fashion accents. Select carefully and they will add to your look of chic. Take your time in selecting frames—there are styles and colors galore. When you find the basic shape that suits your face, try it in several sizes. View yourself in a full length mirror; the frame should be right for your build as well as your face. Heavy frames overpower if you're petite; flimsy ones are out of character if you're tall or big-boned. The frame color should complement your skin tone, hair, wardrobe. Generally, lighter tones are best for pale or pink-toned complexions; deeper tones for olive or darker complexions.

Now for your makeup: With glasses *off,* apply foundation and powder. Brush away excess powder from around the eyes. Use blush lightly on the cheekbones, keeping it below the eyeglass area. In applying lipstick, avoid drawing a pursed, rosebud mouth. Lips with a wider, gently feminine curve create balanced harmony with glasses. Eyebrows must be well-groomed and shouldn't disappear behind the top frame. If necessary, pencil in a little added height to your brow. Extend the brow line to parallel the frame; don't let it droop at the end.

If your lenses magnify, they will tend to intensify the color and effect of eye makeup. Use soft or pastel tones of shadow, preferably matte shadow. Eyeliner should be in charcoal, ash brown, or blue; darker tones will be too harsh. Brown or dark blue mascara is attractive.

Nonmagnifying or tinted lenses diminish eye makeup. They call for a livelier tone of eye shadow, possibly with a little gleam. Eyeliner can be more positive—black or dark brown if you're a brunette; charcoal or soft brown if you're fair. Mascara should be black or dark brown.

Study your eye makeup in a strong light, both with your glasses and without them, to determine the right degree of color for best effect. And remember—you're not hiding behind your glasses. They actually spotlight your eyes, and with beautifully applied makeup, they can enhance your looks.

> *"Dear Miss Rubinstein:*
> *Please advise me about eye makeup with contact lenses. I've been told that if a tiny flake gets under a lens it's very irritating."*

Use a reputable brand of eye makeup and apply it correctly. Then there'll be little chance of a flake getting into your eye. To be extra cautious, however, you might use a creamy shadow rather than the dry, powdery type, and use a mascara formula without the filaments that add thickness. Apply eye shadow and liner *before* you put in *hard* contact lenses. Once they're in, you shouldn't use even the lightest finger pressure across the lid. Shadow and liner can be applied *after soft* contact lenses have been inserted, however (or before, if you prefer). I understand that, as well as being more comfortable for daylong use, soft lenses are less likely to trap any particles (of eye makeup or other matter) underneath them. Lightly tinted contact lenses cut down glare when they're in, and when they're out are easier to find than transparent ones. Contact lenses in colors to match or slightly intensify the iris can be interesting. However, don't choose a shade too far from your eyes' own color; the result can be strange and unnatural. (Note: only hard lenses are available in tints.)

12

The Contemporary
Woman

The world changes. Beauty is no longer its own excuse for being. A perfect shell, an exquisite ornament, a china doll, belong in a glass case. Today's woman doesn't.

There is an awareness abroad in our world today. Eyes are sharper and minds are clearer. There is a closer examination of issues and a reappraisal of philosophies. Smoke screens, sham, pretense, are no longer tolerated with a knowing wink. There is a profound consciousness that this is a pivotal moment in time. And today's woman relates to her time in history. She is alert, alive, informed, involved. She is aware of her appearance, of course. Today's woman cares for her looks with more precision and effectiveness than women of any other generation, yet she spends less time on rituals, wastes less energy on vanity. Beauty is part of her life—not an obsession. Her beauty care is planned to fit neatly into her schedule, and fully confident of her attractive appearance, she then moves on to the important job of living. She doesn't whip out her mirror for frequent checks on her makeup, or poke at her hair, or tug at her clothes. These things were taken care of expertly at the right time—now she's too busy doing other things.

The most attractive women in the world are running households, serving as volunteers in schools and hospitals, assisting in environmental or community programs. They hold jobs of every description; their interests range to every subject. They recognize the world's imperfections, and with their indomitable female instinct for order and beauty they are acting, in ways great and small, to improve our planet.

When I was first in Paris, I heard the Frenchman's timeworn description of the perfect woman (you've heard it, too)—*cuisinière* in the kitchen, *grande dame* in the salon, *maitresse* in the bedroom. Today's woman would find such "perfection" too limiting. She has more versatility than the original Frenchman ever dreamed of. Along with expertise in kitchen, salon, and bedroom, she combines knowledge and skill in the arts, business, politics, sports. If she has children, she also must acquit herself creditably as chauffeur, mediator, psychologist.

It's true that women today are more active, more influential, more competitive than at any other time in history. Yet the outstanding women of our era have retained an enchanting femininity. Some of the most intelligent, vying with men for key positions, are among the most feminine. If they compete with men, it is with their minds and their skills—and they earn more respect and more lasting success as a result. I don't believe women should "use" their sex in business; I don't believe they should *lose* it either. Womanliness is a part of you that belongs in your appearance and your attitude; it needn't be prostituted as an excuse, weapon, or enticement in business.

One of the fascinating things about the contemporary woman of beauty is that she looks just as she should. Her face, her stance, her manner as well as her appearance belong to this moment, and all reflect her essential character. Qualities of mind and spirit may seem intangible, yet they become clearly imprinted on the individual. They are apparent in the glance of an eye, the line of a mouth, the way the head is held or the hand is used. They can be heard in the tone of the voice and its message. They are conveyed by the fragrance a woman has chosen to express her personality. Mental attitude has a most persistent way of translating itself into physical terms. Optimism, empathy, interest, a sense of humor, all leave a lasting mark of beauty.

The most beautiful contemporary women are those who give something of themselves to every occasion—a smile, a laugh, words that spark conversation, but most of all sincere interest in others. One of the most charming women I have ever met is the wife of a famous man and a brilliant writer. She is small, quiet, unpretentious—yet completely unforgettable. Although her own activities are tremendous, she rarely talks of herself. She devotes her full attention to the person she is with—her smile is warm, her eyes dance with interest, she seems utterly absorbed in what the other is saying. Little wonder she captivates all who meet her.

Another woman, the wife of a noted diplomat, is also a "giver." She is a fighter for causes and is constantly involved in worthwhile projects. Because of her verve and animation, one often forgets that she experienced great personal tragedy in the past and, due to a spinal problem that cannot be completely remedied, is often in considerable pain. Self-pity? There isn't a shred in her. In her life there has been a great deal that could depress her—if she would let it. She doesn't. When she enters a room it is suddenly alive, more inviting. She bubbles with humor that lifts the mood of all around her.

Fascinating women who brighten the scene aren't met only at diplomatic balls or elegant soirées. There are many who add a dimension of joy in everyday places—where they work, where they live, wherever they happen to be. What sets these women apart? I think it is their ability to keep things in perspective; to see their own lives in correct relation to those around them; to contribute a "plus" rather than a "minus" to all the lives they touch. These women do not wrap themselves in cocoons of self-interest. They look outside of themselves—and find a world of excitement waiting. They have a natural curiosity on a broad, not a petty, scale; they have a sense of adventure, a *joie de vivre*. They have a lovingness toward people, places, things—and love, we all know, is irresistible.

Charm of manner, an optimistic approach to life, *do* come more easily to some than to others. If you were not so gifted, however, they *can* be developed. Since your personality traits are as much a part of your beauty as your hairstyle and your complexion, they certainly should be given objective scrutiny at frequent intervals. You change your lipstick shade from time to time; you may also need to change your attitude.

Negative thinking can be an insidious thing, building up gradually, often stealthily, and taking over as a very bad habit. Complaining, nagging, backbiting, envy are qualities that bore one's friends and devastate one's looks. Listen to yourself next time you are with a group. If you have fallen into the dreary trap, make a determined effort to improve your mental attitude. Stop airing your complaints. Others have problems, too; perhaps far more serious than yours. Listen more and speak less. Turn your interest outside of yourself. Try to understand others; then try a little harder. Bring your sense of humor out of hiding. Develop a whole new philosophy if necessary.

When you desperately need a change of mind, try a change of pace. A break in routine can give you a fresh start. A new hobby, study, sport, or friend are all "stretchers" that help broaden the mind, add to the joy of living, and eventually make you a far more attractive person.

As I mentioned earlier in this book, happiness is a great contributor to beauty. Throughout my career women have asked me, "How can I be beautiful?" The second most frequently asked question (though it is phrased in a thousand different ways) is, "How can I be happy?" The answer to each question is within oneself. Beauty can be cultivated; any woman who invests a little time and effort can achieve her most attractive appearance. Happiness—a nebulous thing at best—can be attained only when one has come to terms with life itself. It consists not so much in getting everything one wants but rather in enjoying what one gets. There can be delight in the myriad things that make up a day—a child's laugh, the miracle of beauty in a single flower, the glory of the sun, the freshness of the rain, the satisfaction of a project completed whether it be the creation of a delicious meal or a magnificent painting. Indispensable to happiness is sharing—of one's time, one's thoughts, and—of course, of one's beauty!

In each of the many women I have met I have found a unique quality—her own very special beauty, sometimes budding, sometimes blooming, sometimes begging to be nurtured. Helping women to recognize this quality, to polish and perfect it, has been one of the great satisfactions of my life. The greatest pleasure of all will consist in reaching, through these pages, some of you whom I may never have the opportunity to meet in person. From this mélange of instruction, thoughts and reminiscences, I hope you will extract many ideas for your *own* beauty and the inspiration to apply them faithfully. It has been a joy for me to share with you, and along with beauty, I wish you many happy tomorrows.

Index

Cheeks:
  applying color to, 49-50
  contour treatment for, 33
  "French Facial Gymnastics"
    for, 35
Chest, exercise for, 119-20, 130
Chin:
  contour treatment for, 32
  double, makeup and, 65
  "French Facial Gymnastics"
    for, 35
  plastic surgery for, 220
  receding, makeup and, 64
Circulation of blood, skin and, 29
Clothes, see Dress
Coffee, 92-93
  in underweight diet, 111
Cologne, 162, 163
Color rinse, 176
Combination skin, see Skin,
  combination
Complexion, see Skin
Conditioning of hair, 169-70, 187
  with treated hair, 178
Contact lenses, 36
  makeup and, 228
Contour treatment, 29-34
Corrective plastic surgery, 220
Cosmetic masks, 27-29
Cosmetics:
  cost of, 226-27
  natural vs. commercial, 225-56
  See also Makeup
"Crash" diets, 96-97
Curling hair, 179
Cuticle care, 149
Cream rinse, 170

Dancing as relaxation exercise,
  135
"Day of Beauty":
  at Helena Rubinstein Salon,
    207-11
  at home, 212-14
Dental care, 85, 157
Deodorants, 157

Depilation:
  of arms, 147-48
  facial, 40-41
  of legs, 153-54
Dermis, definition of, 3
Derriere, exercise for, 125
"Detractors", 48-49
Diaphragm, exercise for, 120
Dieting, 94-116
  "crash", 96-97
  general remarks on, 94-97,
    115-16
  and ideal-weight maintenance,
    104-5
  "Ten Commandments of
    Slimming", 97-98
  Three-Step Reducing Plan,
    98-104
  for weight gain, 110-15
  working woman's lunch,
    108-10
  Zig-Zag Diet, 105-8
  See also Nutrition
Dowager's hump, 122, 128, 138,
  189
Dress, 197-204
  color and, 202-4
  fashion organizer (chart), 200
  fashion trends and, 197-98
  mature women and, 189-92
  total look in, 199-202
Drugs:
  appetite suppressants, 96
  and skin, 5
Dusting powder, 162

Ears:
  care of, 158
  plastic surgery and, 220
Elbow care, 146-47
Electrolysis, 40-41
Emotions and skin, 4, 5, 18
Epidermis, definition of, 3
Evening, makeup for, 47, 69-72
Exercise(s), 85, 116-38
  basic daily, 121-26